GOING VEGAN FOR BEGINNERS

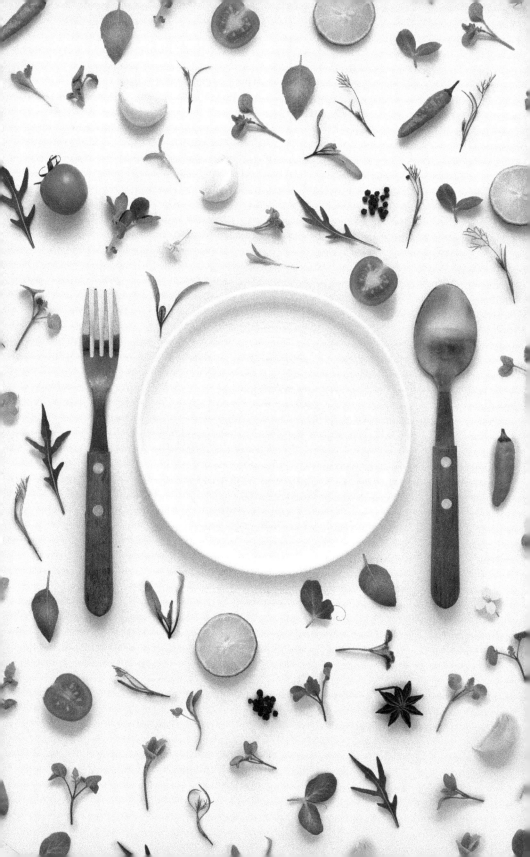

GOING VEGAN
FOR BEGINNERS

THE ESSENTIAL NUTRITION GUIDE TO
TRANSITIONING TO A VEGAN DIET

PAMELA FERGUSSON, RD, PHD

ROCKRIDGE
PRESS

Interior and Cover Designer: Lisa Forde
Art Producer: Meg Baggott
Editor: Van Van Cleave
Production Editors: Rachel Taenzler, Jax Berman
Production Manager: Riley Hoffman

Photography © Peiling Lee/Shutterstock, ii; Darren Muir, vi; Foxys Forest Manufacture/Shutterstock, x; Oksana Mizina/Shutterstock, 12; tanya_morozz/Shutterstock, 24; Rimma Bondarenko/Shutterstock, 42; SherSor/Shutterstock, 54; StudioPhotoDFlorez/Shutterstock, 66; ILEISH ANNA/Shutterstock, 80; Nina Firsova/Shutterstock, 92; Andrew Purcell, 103; Fortyforks/Shutterstock, 104; Sea Wave/Shutterstock, 112; Thomas J. Story, 127; Laura Flippen; 128.
Author photo courtesy of Trista Verhesen /Authentic Living Photography.

Paperback ISBN: 978-1-64876-660-2 | eBook ISBN: 978-1-64876-159-1
R0

FOR MY CHILDREN,
Bly, Cedar, Willow, and Fern,
who inspire me to be better.
For René, who believed in
me. For my parents, who
called every day to see how
the writing was going. And,
as always, for the animals.

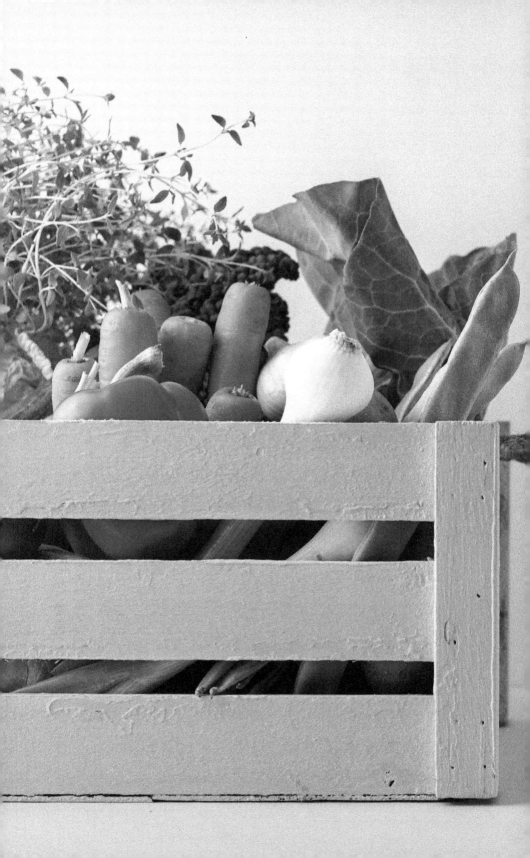

CONTENTS

INTRODUCTION

I spend every day helping individuals and families optimize their health with plants. I'm a registered dietitian, and veganism has been the focus of my nutrition practice since 2014. As an expert in the field, I am pleased to be able to write a book sharing my knowledge with you as you embark on your journey to build a healthy vegan diet.

While I was studying nutrition in college, I read a book called *Diet for a Small Planet* by Frances Moore Lappé. I learned that we have enough food in the world to feed everyone; we just need to distribute that food differently, feeding plant calories directly to humans instead of to animals in the animal agriculture industry. That book inspired me to go vegetarian. It was an easy transition for me because I had always loved animals and I never liked the idea of eating them. I can remember being so upset as a child when my cousin shot a few rounds over the heads of some crows who were eating grain in my uncle's fields. He was only trying to scare the birds, but I didn't like thinking of animals being shot.

When I decided to open my private practice as a dietitian, I began deeply researching the relationship between personal health and nutrition in North America. I was aware that Canadians and Americans were facing an epidemic of cancer, diabetes, heart disease, and high blood pressure, and I wanted to offer my clients a way to prevent these diseases and optimize their health. In my research, I discovered that eating a plant-based diet can reduce the risk of disease and increase longevity. I was convinced!

I went completely plant-based myself, first for just 30 days. I found it easy, and I felt good, so I kept going. I had worried about giving up cheese, but I found vegan food to be so satisfying and delicious that my cravings soon went away. Not long after going vegan, I watched some shocking videos about animal agriculture. After I understood the impact of animal agriculture on the planet and saw the mistreatment of animals, I committed to being vegan for life.

Your decision to go vegan probably reflects many of the things that influenced me. Veganism is growing as a movement for many good reasons. People are going vegan because they know it is better for the planet, better for the animals, and better for their personal health. I could write a whole book about *why* to go vegan, but this book is on *how* to go vegan, with a focus on personal health benefits. Whether you are already vegan, interested in going vegan, or looking to optimize your health by eating more plants and less meat, this book covers everything you need to know.

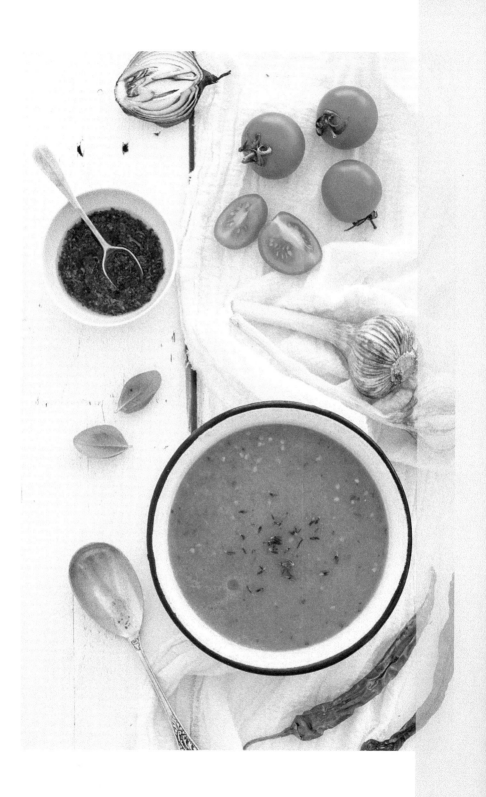

CHAPTER 1

WHAT IS THE VEGAN DIET AND WHY SHOULD I TRY IT?

The first step to creating and following a nutritious and delicious vegan diet is understanding what veganism is and how it differs from other dietary approaches, such as vegetarian and plant-based diets. This chapter explores the meaning of veganism, its social justice aspects, and its health benefits. I also define other related dietary approaches to provide helpful context for your new lifestyle.

Veganism Defined

Veganism is a philosophy and way of life that extends far beyond diet. The Vegan Society defines veganism as "a way of living that seeks to exclude, as far as possible and practicable, all forms of exploitation of, and cruelty to, animals for food, clothing, and any other purpose." Veganism is a social justice issue, and underpinning that issue is a belief that animals have rights, and their bodies are not ours to exploit.

In general, vegans practice a lifestyle that encourages protection and respect for the rights of species other than our own. This practice is in contrast to the idea of speciesism. In his book *Animal Liberation,* Peter Singer defined speciesism as "a prejudice or attitude of bias in favor of the interests of members of one's own species and against those of members of other species." Speciesism has its origins in the view that humans are the apex of life on Earth and animals are here to serve the needs of humans. Speciesism also relates to how humans classify the value of different species of animals—treating their family dog much better than they would treat a pig raised for pork, for example.

Within the veganism movement, there are a variety of approaches and schools of thought. The following sections provide a brief introduction to some of the primary concerns and debates within the larger movement. I invite you to participate in discussions and do your own research if you are interested in diving deeper into any of the positions mentioned here.

VEGAN ACTIVISM

Vegan activists are people who advocate for animal rights and promote veganism. Activism can take many forms, including hosting vegan potlucks, political campaigns, protests, sharing vegan food ideas on social media, or speaking about veganism with family and friends. Activists are motivated by the fact that there are about 77 billion land animals slaughtered for food each year, and those animals cannot advocate for themselves. The scale and urgency of the problem motivates some vegans to advocate exclusively for the rights of animals.

ANTI-OPPRESSION FRAMEWORK VS. ANIMALS-FIRST APPROACH

An anti-oppression framework means that to oppose any form of oppression, we must oppose all forms of oppression. Vegans, including myself, who take this approach bring animal rights to the anti-oppression discussion table. This increased awareness of the plight of animals, and the act of asking advocates from other social justice backgrounds to recognize the rights of animals, helps expand those rights. In turn, vegan activists can uphold the rights of people from oppressed groups both within and outside the vegan movement.

Contrary to the anti-oppression framework, vegans who take an animals-first approach believe that vegan activists should focus solely on bringing attention to the oppression that animals face, and let other social justice causes advocate for themselves.

ABOLITIONISM VS. ANIMAL WELFARE

Vegans differ on the best approach to achieving animal liberation. Some vegans believe in taking an abolitionist approach, which means they would advocate only for the total liberation of animals, and not accept a step-by-step approach to achieving this. Other vegans take a more pragmatic approach of advocating for improvements in the conditions animals endure in the animal agriculture industry, on the way to achieving full liberation. Campaigns to abolish gestation crates for pigs or battery cages for hens are examples of animal-welfare campaigns. Personally, I believe in advocating for animal liberation, but I also recognize we are a long way from a vegan world. I take an animal-welfare approach and believe in improving conditions for the billions of animals currently living in oppressive conditions due to animal agriculture.

CRUELTY-FREE LABELS

"Cruelty-free" is a term you may see on labels for cosmetics, foods, or household products, and the term is a source of some confusion. When you see terms such as "cruelty-free" and "vegan" on labels, the differences in meaning are not always clear. "Cruelty-free" is commonly used in the cosmetics industry to indicate that a product has not been tested on animals. This term is somewhat problematic because it is possible for a cosmetic product not to be tested on animals, but still contain animal products and, therefore, not be vegan. The term "cruelty-free" also does not consider the human labor abuses that are often problematic in the cosmetics industry, and that fact is true for food products as well because even fruit and vegetable production commonly involve poor working conditions for migrant farm laborers. If you have doubts about the products you purchase, the best practice is to do your own research, rather than rely on potentially misleading labels.

The Vegan Diet

As you can see, veganism extends beyond diet. However, this book specifically focuses on the nutrition principles of a vegan diet—the dietary part of veganism.

Vegans exclude all animal products from their diets. Although a vegan diet can consist of predominately or even exclusively whole plant foods, there is an increasing variety of vegan "comfort food" products, such as meat alternatives and vegan ice-cream bars available. Although these "comfort foods" may not be as healthy as whole plants, they are vegan and can be part of a balanced vegan diet.

In this book, I discuss a vegan diet that contains no animal products and is mostly made up of whole plant foods. This is the way I eat, and this way of eating can offer many environmental, ethical, and health benefits while still allowing for some vegan treats. When I refer to a vegan diet, I mean the dietary pattern that vegans follow.

Now that I've defined what a vegan diet is, I think it is also important to define what it is not. It is not a diet in the sense of an eating plan designed for weight loss. Although many people do lose weight as a result of going vegan and changing their eating pattern, not all do, and it is important to recognize that the goal of veganism is animal liberation, not weight loss. And, veganism extends far beyond eating habits. Vegans do not use leather products, for example, or ride horses or go to zoos. But this is a nutrition book, so our focus will be on how to build a healthy way of eating that contains no animal products.

HOW TO EAT A VEGAN DIET TO PROMOTE YOUR HEALTH

There are many ways to eat as a vegan. Some vegans may eat mostly smoothies, salads, protein bowls, and avocado toast. Other vegans may eat a lot of stir-fries, tacos, oatmeal, pizza, pasta, burritos, and burgers. There is an infinite variety of food and meal combinations that vegans can eat, and nearly all cultural dietary patterns can be adapted to be vegan. One of the greatest discoveries of going vegan is the abundance of the plant kingdom and everything it offers for humans to enjoy.

Though there are many ways to eat healthy as a vegan, there are a few principles that all healthy vegan diets have in common:

Eat mostly whole or minimally processed plant foods.

Eat a wide variety of plant-based foods, including fruits and vegetables, nuts and seeds, plant-based proteins, and starches and grains. (We will talk about meeting your nutrient needs in chapters 4 through 7.)

Eat enough to meet your individual needs for optimal health and activity.

BENEFITS OF A VEGAN DIET

You've picked up this book, so I know you have an interest in a vegan diet, which means you may be familiar with some of the many benefits of practicing a vegan diet. These benefits include:

COMPASSIONATE APPROACH

One of the greatest benefits of following a vegan diet is the awareness that you no longer support an oppressive industry that kills 77 billion land animals each year. Veganism can fit into and expand upon an anti-oppression and compassionate approach to life. Be aware, however, that once you are mindful of animals' suffering, that empathy can also bring sadness and overwhelming feelings into your life. Be compassionate with yourself as well.

ENVIRONMENTALLY FRIENDLY

A vegan diet uses less water and less land and produces fewer greenhouse gasses than the standard North American diet. I often get asked, "If everyone went vegan, where would we get the land to grow all the beans, fruits, grains, and vegetables people would need?" What those asking don't realize is that animal agriculture is a much more land-intensive way of producing calories and protein for humans. Most animals grown for food eat grains and, sometimes, soy. Growing those crops for animal feed takes a lot of land—land that could be used to grow alternative foods for humans.

Animals eat far more calories than they produce as food, so raising animals is not an efficient way of creating food for humans. The efficiency looks slightly better for animals raised on land that would otherwise not be appropriate for growing food for humans (for example, much of the arid land in the western United States). However, these animals represent a small proportion of meat sold in North America. Pasture-raised meat tends to be more expensive, and we would not be able to raise enough of it to meet demand.

A diet high in animal products tends to have a much higher water and greenhouse gas footprint than a vegan diet as well.

A lot of this footprint comes from the methane produced directly by animals raised for meat. A significant portion of the environmental impact also comes from the water used and greenhouse gas emissions created by growing the feed used to raise animals for food. Vegans can further shrink their footprint by eating fewer highly processed foods and eating local and in season.

HEALTHIER MICROBIOME

Your microbiome is made up of the bacteria that live in your gut. Building a healthier microbiome is one of the greatest benefits of adopting a healthy vegan diet. Healthy bacteria need fiber to survive, and fiber only comes from plants. In addition to promoting a healthy gut, a high-fiber diet also helps prevent diabetes, heart disease, hypertension, and some cancers. Surprisingly, only about 5 percent of people in the United States meet their recommended fiber intake goals.

Your microbiome plays a big role in shaping your mental health as well as your physical health. Improving gut health can reduce your risk of developing depression, improve digestion, and help ward off infection. Research into the microbiome is among the hottest topics in medicine at the moment, and new discoveries are being made all the time. Even though we are still learning a lot about the human microbiome, there is no doubt that feeding your gut bacteria with healthy, whole plant foods is one of the best things you can do for your overall health.

IMPROVED INSULIN SENSITIVITY

Insulin is a hormone that enables your body to convert glucose into energy. If you develop insulin resistance, which means your cells do not respond properly to insulin, your blood sugar level will increase and your body will continue to produce more and more insulin to try to regulate it. Eventually, your pancreas can become damaged, and you may develop type 2 diabetes as well as an increased risk for heart attack, kidney disease, and stroke.

Insulin resistance, also called metabolic syndrome, is incredibly common: About one-third of the population of the United States has insulin resistance. The good news is that insulin sensitivity can improve. Adopting a healthy vegan diet, exercising more, getting adequate sleep, and reducing stress are all good strategies for improving insulin sensitivity.

LOWER BLOOD LIPIDS

Cholesterol and triglycerides are fats found in your blood and tissues. Having high levels of triglycerides and cholesterol can create a buildup of these fats in your artery walls, which can lead to increased risk of heart disease and stroke. Heart disease is the leading cause of death in the United States, and stroke is number five.

One of the best ways to reduce these health risks is to eat a fiber-rich vegan diet. Fiber is a particularly important part of a cholesterol-lowering diet, and fiber is only found in plant foods. Activity, healthy diet, and stress reduction can all help lower blood lipids as well.

Vegetarianism and Other Plant-Based Diets

The vegan diet shares some similarities with other popular dietary patterns, such as vegetarianism and plant-based eating. Given these similarities and the overlap with some of these eating patterns, it can be tricky to understand where one ends and another begins. The following information should help.

VEGETARIANISM

In most cases, the term "vegetarian" means "lacto-ovo vegetarian," which is a person who eats vegan foods along with dairy, eggs, and honey. The same word, "vegetarian," is used to describe the person and the food item, such as a vegetarian omelet or vegetarian pizza. You might also see it shortened to "veggie" on menus—veggie burger, for example.

Vegetarian foods never contain meat or fish. And a product or menu item labeled vegetarian may, in fact, be vegan if it contains no dairy, eggs, or honey. If you see a product or menu item labeled vegetarian, read the ingredients label or ask whether it contains nonvegan items, such as dairy products, eggs, or honey.

Although vegetarians may feel aligned with vegans because neither eat meat or fish, many vegans feel that the dairy and egg industries are some of the cruelest in the animal agriculture industry. In her 1990 book *The Sexual Politics of Meat*, Carol J. Adams points out that the female reproductive systems of cows and chickens are repeatedly exploited in the dairy and egg industries.

Many people are unaware, for example, that dairy cows produce milk only after being impregnated through artificial insemination, and when they give birth, their calves are removed from them so the farmers can take the milk to sell for human consumption. Male calves are fattened and sold as veal, whereas females are raised to join their mothers in milk production. Once hens and cows have passed peak production, they are killed. Many vegetarians are attracted to the diet because they don't want to contribute to animal suffering or death, but the dairy industry is the veal industry, and all animals in the animal agriculture industry are eventually slaughtered.

PLANT-BASED DIET

"Plant-based diet" is a phrase that can mean several things. "Plant-based" usually indicates a product or meal is made completely from plants, but it can also mean it's made predominantly from plants. It's important to be careful when buying products labeled "plant-based"—read the ingredients label. Some products labeled "plant-based" may actually contain animal products, such as dairy or eggs.

Similarly, someone who says they follow a plant-based diet may mean they eat only plant-based foods and consume no animal products, but they may also mean they are eating

predominantly plant-based and that they occasionally consume animal products. In some cases, people may decide to be
plant-based at home but eat animal products when dining in
restaurants or while a guest in someone else's home. Others may
eat plant-based for breakfast and lunch and then, sometimes,
include animal products with their evening meal.

Most people who use the term "plant-based" are interested
primarily in the health benefits of a vegan diet, though they may
not identify as vegan, even if they completely avoid eating animal
products, because the ethical arguments for veganism may not
resonate. Also, someone who is plant-based may or may not avoid
cleaning products, clothing, cosmetics, or entertainment that uses
animals.

Most people who eat a plant-based diet for health reasons
choose whole food options most of the time and avoid or limit
their intake of vegan comfort food products, such as vegan sausages and ice cream. Many people start following a plant-based
diet because they are attracted to the health benefits, and then
become aware of the environmental and ethical dilemmas we face
in our food system, and eventually become vegan. Not everyone
does, however—some people maintain a plant-based diet and
never become vegan.

WHOLE FOODS PLANT-BASED DIET

In the term "whole foods plant-based," each word has a meaning,
and the meaning is exactly as it sounds. "Whole foods" means
foods that are unadulterated or minimally processed and include
beans, fruits, grains, lentils, nuts and seeds, tempeh, tofu, and, of
course, vegetables. Veggies and fruits can be fresh or frozen and
beans can be cooked from dried or canned, and minimally processed foods, such as tofu, are okay, but more highly processed
foods, such as commercial vegan sausages or burgers, are not
considered whole foods. Oil is considered processed and is not
included in the whole foods plant-based eating pattern.

"Plant-based" means the foods should be of plant origin.
Most proponents of the whole foods plant-based way of life

promote eating only plant-based foods, whereas some say eating plant-based 90 to 95 percent of the time is acceptable, with some low-fat animal products included.

Whole foods plant-based eating is a high-fiber, high-volume, low-caloric-density way of eating. The concept is that you can eat as much food as you are hungry for, as long as the foods are whole foods and plant-based. Some people choose to eat a high-starch diet, focusing on potatoes, sweet potatoes, and whole grains, complemented by nonstarchy vegetables, with some fruit and small portions of nuts and seeds. Others take a more balanced approach, aiming to fill half their plate with fruits and veggies and make up the balance with grains, nuts and seeds, plant-based proteins, and starches.

People eating a whole foods plant-based diet typically eat a low-fat diet, which is mostly a natural result of eating whole plant foods and eliminating oils. Some leaders of the whole foods plant-based movement encourage followers to limit avocado, coconut, and nuts and seeds to keep fat intake low, even when it comes from whole plant foods.

Many people following the whole foods plant-based diet have experienced dramatic health improvements, including improved blood sugar control, reduced cholesterol levels, and normalized blood pressure. It's important to note, however, that this way of eating will not suit everyone, and the effects on each individual's health will vary. The whole foods plant-based diet is a way of life that many people love and become devoted to, but others may find it too extreme or restrictive, and some don't get the results they expected.

It is possible to gain health benefits from going vegan without being fully whole foods plant-based, especially if you don't suffer from chronic sickness and your goals are to optimize health and prevent disease.

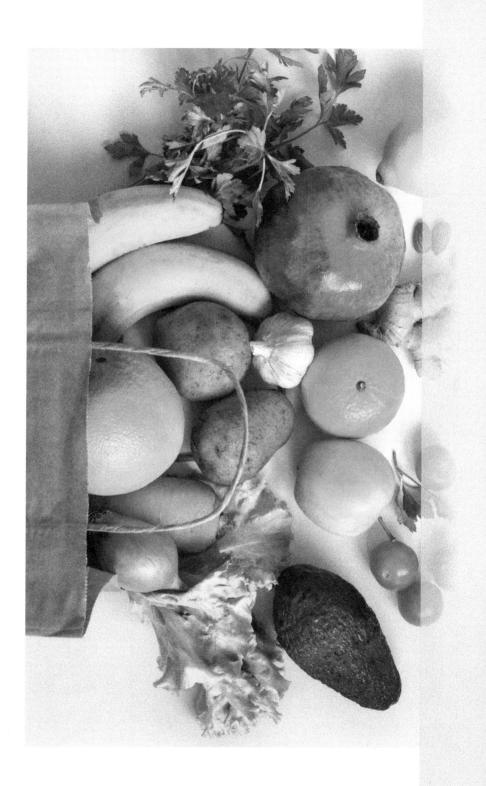

CHAPTER 2

COMPLETE NUTRITION AND THE HEALTH BENEFITS OF A VEGAN DIET

There is no single perfect diet that can guarantee good health. However, diet does have a huge impact on our health. The standard North American diet, which is high in ultra-processed foods, sugar, and salt, is a major contributor to premature death and disability, whereas a healthy vegan diet can reduce your risk of developing the diseases that are the most common killers in North America.

A completely plant-based diet can help you optimize your health and reduce your risk of chronic disease—from reducing inflammation to lowering the risk of diabetes, heart disease, and stroke. In this chapter, we'll explore these health benefits.

Obesity

Obesity is defined as a body mass index (BMI) of 30 or greater. According to the most recent data from the Centers for Disease Control and Prevention (CDC), about 42 percent of US adults are obese. Obesity can lead to many health complications, including gallbladder disease, gout, nonalcoholic fatty liver disease, and type 2 diabetes.

Before we dive into the ways that a vegan diet can support healthy weight loss, it's important to address some questions regarding the concept of obesity as a disease. BMI was never intended to be an individual diagnostic tool; that is, it was not meant to be used on its own to determine whether someone is healthy. BMI works best as a tool when combined with other factors and measurements. BMI is prone to errors (especially when people are very tall or very short) and tends to misclassify muscular people as overweight or obese. Furthermore, the BMI standard was developed using data only from white European people and, so, is not well adapted for use with people from other racial and ethnic backgrounds. There is also an increasing body of literature documenting the negative impact of anti-fatness in health care and in society, and on the increased risks of death and disease associated with weight cycling and internalized fatphobia.

To address these concerns, the Health at Every Size movement offers a different perspective on weight. Health at Every Size does not mean that every person is healthy at every weight, but rather that every person has the right to pursue health, regardless of size. By shifting the focus to improving blood work, fitness, intuitive eating, mental health, and quality of life, and away from the number on the scale, Health at Every Size practitioners encourage people to find more compassionate ways to take care of themselves. Health at Every Size also calls into question the notion that personal health choices are the most important determinant of health and, instead, acknowledges that individual genetic factors and systemic race and class structures can also affect body size.

The Health at Every Size movement offers a more robust and well-rounded approach to promoting health. The important takeaway from this approach is that your health is about more than a number on the scale. If you have concerns about your weight, consider speaking with a health-care provider about your concerns as they relate to your health (both physical and mental) as well as your quality of life.

Even with the understanding that BMI is not a perfect indicator of health, research regarding BMI demonstrates that a vegan diet can help prevent obesity and related health concerns. The Adventist Health Study-2, for example, followed 96,000 members of the Seventh-day Adventist Church in Canada and the United States. Researchers reported that vegans had the lowest BMIs, with a mean BMI of 24.1; lacto-ovo vegetarians were next, at a BMI of 26.1. The average BMI for nonvegetarians was 28.3. This was an observational study, which means that participants were not asked to change their diets in any way, only to report on what they were already doing.

Studies such as this one demonstrate that a healthy vegan diet that is high in fiber and based mostly on whole foods may be helpful in achieving and maintaining a healthy body weight. There are other effective measures for maintaining a healthy body weight, including focusing on filling half your plate with fruits and vegetables, choosing whole grains, eating only when you are hungry and stopping when you are full, moving your body in a way that feels good to you, staying hydrated, and prioritizing sleep and stress management.

Inflammation

Inflammation is the body's process of responding to perceived potential harm, which could be from infection, injury, or toxins. The body will attempt to heal itself by producing a cascade of reactions from the immune system. That response to harm is wonderful if you are trying to fight off an acute infection for a few days, but, sometimes, this immune response can linger, leaving your body in a heightened state of stress for months, or even years. This condition is chronic inflammation, and it can lead to increased risk of disease.

Chronic inflammation can come from many sources in our lives, and a healthy diet, along with activity, sleep, and stress reduction, can help reduce inflammation. No single individual food significantly contributes to or reduces inflammation; instead, inflammation is a function of our overall dietary pattern. A healthy vegan diet is naturally anti-inflammatory.

Reducing your intake of sugars from foods such as commercial cakes, doughnuts, sweets, deep-fried foods, processed meats, and sugar-sweetened beverages will help reduce inflammation. In place of these inflammatory foods, a vegan diet fills your plate with fruits and vegetables, nuts and seeds, whole grains, and plant-based proteins such as beans, lentils, and soy. Berries, chia seeds, flaxseed, garlic, ginger, greens, turmeric, and walnuts, all rich in omega-3 fatty acids, may be particularly helpful in reducing inflammation. Following this anti-inflammatory dietary pattern will help improve overall health and reduce risk factors for chronic disease.

Stroke

A stroke occurs when the blood supply to a part of your brain is reduced or interrupted. Within minutes, your brain cells start dying. Strokes may occur when there is a clot or a blockage in a blood vessel in the brain, usually because of plaque buildup on artery walls. Strokes may also occur when an artery in the brain breaks open. This breakage can occur because of high blood pressure, which, over time, leads to weakened artery walls that become more vulnerable to breakage.

A diet rich in fruits and vegetables and low in salt and added sugars is helpful in preventing strokes, and a vegan diet naturally includes many foods that are beneficial in maintaining normal blood pressure and a healthy circulatory system. Omega-3-rich chia seeds, flaxseed, and walnuts, along with tomatoes, are useful for stroke prevention, as are foods high in potassium, such as bananas, spinach, and sweet potatoes. Avoid calcium supplements, as they can increase the risk of stroke.

Diabetes

People who have diabetes cannot effectively process food into energy. The hormone insulin helps regulate blood sugar and brings it into cells for energy. When people become resistant to insulin, the pancreas will produce more and more of it to try to regulate blood sugar. Eventually, if the body is not able to keep blood sugar within a normal range, diabetes results.

In the United States, about 13 percent of adults have diabetes, and this rate is on the rise; in 1990 that figure was 5 percent. Diabetes is a disease with multiple risk factors, which include family history; living in poverty; being of African American, Native North American, or South Asian ethnicity; older age; sedentary lifestyle; poor diet; polycystic ovary syndrome; depression; a history of gestational diabetes; high blood pressure; and high triglycerides or cholesterol. Some of these risk factors are within our individual control, and some are not.

Fortunately, research indicates that a vegan diet can help reduce the risk of diabetes. In 2009, Dr. Neal Barnard, adjunct associate professor of medicine at the George Washington University School of Medicine in Washington, DC, and president of the Physicians Committee for Responsible Medicine, published a study that compared the effectiveness of two diets in patients with type 2 diabetes. In his study, 49 people with type 2 diabetes were randomly assigned a low-fat vegan diet, and 50 people were randomly assigned a diet that followed the American Diabetes Association (ADA) guidelines. At the end of the 74-week trial, the participants who ate the vegan diet had lost more weight, had improved blood glucose control, and had greater reductions in blood cholesterol than those who ate the ADA diet.

The message is clear: Eating a healthy vegan diet can help prevent diabetes and can also be a successful diet for managing diabetes. There are several key factors of the vegan diet that make it well suited for those with type 2 diabetes: the type of carbo-hydrates eaten, choosing plant rather than animal proteins, and eating unsaturated fats rather than saturated or trans fats (see chapter 6 for a more detailed discussion of the types of fats).

The evidence includes more than that single study, though. A review of 13 clinical trials published in the journal *Nutrients* in 2015 found that, across all trials, replacing animal proteins with plant proteins improved blood glucose control. This improvement was true even when plant proteins replaced only 35 percent of the animal proteins in the diet.

The choice of fats is also an important factor in preventing and managing diabetes. In fact, there are many relevant dietary factors, and fat intake is one of them. Greater consumption of sat-urated and trans fats—fats found in animal-based foods and highly processed foods—increases the risk of developing diabetes.

An innovative study published in 2003 in *The American Journal of Clinical Nutrition* confirmed this connection by analyzing the blood of almost 3,000 adults and recording the types of fats pres-ent. Researchers then monitored participants for nine years to see who would develop diabetes. Those with higher intakes and blood levels of saturated fats (mostly from animal sources) were signifi-cantly more likely to develop diabetes, whereas the presence of unsaturated fats (from vegetable sources) did not increase the risk of diabetes. This finding is very important, especially given the cur-rent trend to replace carbohydrate intake with fat. In fact, increased intake of saturated fats increases the risk of diabetes.

In the standard North American diet, saturated fat comes mostly from animal products such as dairy, eggs, and meat. A healthy vegan diet is naturally low in saturated fats and high in fiber. Beans, lentils, nuts and seeds, and soy foods all contribute to improved glucose control, as well as lower cholesterol, tri-glycerides, and blood pressure. The fiber in plant-based proteins contributes to a healthier microbiome. This overall picture of better health and reduced risk is beneficial for those looking to prevent or manage type 2 diabetes.

High Blood Pressure

Blood pressure is a way of measuring how hard your heart has to work to pump blood throughout your body. High blood pressure, or hypertension, is widespread and dangerous. It is a risk factor for developing other diseases, including heart disease and stroke. People with diabetes are twice as likely to develop high blood pressure, demonstrating how chronic diseases "cluster."

Nearly half of adults in the United States (45 percent) have high blood pressure (defined as above $\frac{130}{80}$ mmHg), but only about one-fourth of those have their hypertension under control. The CDC reported that, in 2018, nearly half a million deaths in America had hypertension as a primary or contributing cause.

Thankfully, a healthy vegan diet can go a long way to preventing or controlling high blood pressure. Once again, the Adventist Health Study-2 provides evidence for this fact. The study reported that vegans and lacto-ovo vegetarians were significantly less likely to have hypertension than non-vegetarians. Vegans had the lowest risk. This finding was also borne out in the EPIC-Oxford study, which looked at a British population. In this study, when comparing meat eaters, pescatarians (those who eat fish but no meat), vegans, and vegetarians, vegans had the lowest prevalence of high blood pressure.

Eating a diet high in fiber can lower your risk of developing high blood pressure, or even help reduce high blood pressure if you already have it. Raw fruit may be particularly useful, but all types of fiber found in beans and lentils, vegetables, nuts and seeds, and whole grains can help reduce blood pressure. Vegan hibiscus tea also has blood pressure–lowering properties, and may be as effective as medication when consumed regularly.

Cancer

No diet can guarantee protection against cancer, but a plant-based diet can reduce your risks. In their landmark book, *The China Study,* Dr. T. Colin Campbell (a nutritional biochemist from

Cornell University) and his son, Dr. Thomas M. Campbell (founder and co-director of the University of Rochester Medicine/Highland Hospital Nutrition in Medicine Research Center) reported on 20 years of data from the China-Cornell-Oxford project, a study that looked at mortality rates and their causes among people living all over China. The study found links between the intake of animal products and disease, including heart disease and diabetes, but also bowel, breast, and prostate cancers. This book was influential in starting the whole food plant-based dietary trend, and it remains a key text for that movement.

The China Study is not alone in linking diet and cancer. In 2015, the World Health Organization (WHO) claimed headlines around the world with its announcement that consumption of processed meat is "carcinogenic to humans" and that consumption of red meat is "probably carcinogenic to humans." This statement was based on a report written by 22 scientists from 10 countries evaluating more than 800 studies.

The Canadian and American Cancer Societies both recommend healthy diets rich in plants. The Canadian Population Attributable Risk of Cancer (ComPARe) study looked at correlations among behaviors, traits, and exposures in the Canadian population and associated cancer risk. This study reported that alcohol consumption, excess weight, low fruit and vegetable consumption, meat and processed meat consumption, physical inactivity, and smoking were all nutrition- and lifestyle-related factors that increase cancer risk. Based on this data, the Canadian Cancer Society recommends that Canadians eat plenty of fruits and vegetables, whole grains, and plant-based protein foods.

Similarly, the American Cancer Society's Diet and Activity Guidelines state that one in five cases of cancer are caused by lifestyle factors, such as excessive drinking, physical inactivity, and poor diet, and that nutritional factors can increase the risk of 13 types of cancer. The guidelines recommend eating beans and peas, fruits and vegetables, and whole grains. They recommend limiting or avoiding highly processed foods, red and processed meats, sugar-sweetened beverages, and refined grains.

Heart Disease

Globally, heart disease is the leading cause of death. There are many risk factors for heart disease. Some factors you can modify, treat, or control, whereas others you cannot. Your age, being a male, certain ethnicities, having a family history of heart disease, and socioeconomic status are all factors we have little control over. Eating a poor diet, including one with a high alcohol intake; having diabetes, high blood cholesterol and triglycerides, high blood pressure, or a larger waist circumference; physical inactivity; stress; and smoking are all risk factors we can control.

There is strong evidence that a healthy diet can improve heart health. One example of this comes from the documentary *Forks Over Knives*, which shares the work of cardiologist Dr. Caldwell Esselstyn Jr., who directs the Heart Disease Reversal Program at the Cleveland Clinic Wellness & Preventive Medicine Institute. Esselstyn reported on a group of 11 patients who followed a whole food plant-based, no-oil, low-fat diet for at least five years, and were able to see dramatic reductions in their cholesterol levels. These patients all had severe cardiac disease at the start of the study. No one who stuck with the diet for a decade had additional cardiac events.

These results are impressive. However, it should be noted that Esselstyn started with 22 patients, 11 dropped out after 5 years, and only 6 stuck with the diet for the entire 10 years. The high drop-out rate is a criticism that has been leveled at Esselstyn as well as at the whole food plant-based lifestyle in general. Other doctors wonder if it is realistic to ask patients to follow this way of eating. To this criticism, Esselstyn famously, and rather dramatically, replied, "Some people think a plant-based, whole foods diet is extreme. Half a million people a year will have their chests opened up and a vein taken from their leg and sewn onto their coronary artery. Some people would call that extreme."

For those looking to prevent heart disease, you can reduce your risk by eating a diet rich in fiber from whole plant foods;

foods particularly helpful in reducing heart disease risk include apples, barley, beans and lentils, citrus fruits, nuts and seeds, oats and oat bran, soy foods, and strawberries. Psyllium husk is a powerful cholesterol reducer (my favorite way to eat it is mixed into applesauce).

Reducing your intake of, or eliminating, deep-fried foods, foods high in sodium and/or added sugars, and highly processed foods will also help reduce your heart disease risk. The American Heart Association recommends that the average person keeps saturated fat intake to 5 to 6 percent of overall calories, or about 13 grams of saturated fat, or fewer, each day, which is easily done on a healthy vegan diet, as plants are naturally very low in saturated fat. When eating animal products, it is easy to exceed these guidelines. For example, there are about 16 grams of saturated fat in one quarter-pound beef hamburger on a bun served with mayo, ketchup, mustard, and a slice of American cheese, and about 14 grams of saturated fat in a two-egg Western omelet served with ¾ cup of hash browns.

Alzheimer's Disease

About one-third (34.6 percent) of people in the United States age 85 and older have Alzheimer's disease, according to the Alzheimer's Association. This chronic neurogenerative disease causes brain cells to degrade over time. Dr. Dean Sherzai and Dr. Ayesha Sherzai, co-directors of the Alzheimer's Prevention Program at Loma Linda University and authors of *The Alzheimer's Solution*, have a five-part plan that they say will dramatically reduce the risk of developing Alzheimer's disease. One central pillar of their plan is nutrition—specifically, following a plant-based diet that's low in added sugar, salt, and highly processed foods. Their plan for a balanced and healthy lifestyle also includes guidance for exercising, unwinding, resting, and being socially active.

This plan shows that many areas of lifestyle are important in preventing Alzheimer's disease; nutrition is one key intervention. Other approaches also emphasize the efficacy of a plant-based diet in helping prevent Alzheimer's. The MIND diet (Mediterranean-DASH

Intervention for Neurodegenerative Delay) was developed by Dr. Martha Clare Morris and is a hybrid of the Mediterranean diet and the Dietary Approach to Stop Hypertension (DASH) diet. The MIND diet has been shown to slow cognitive decline and reduce the risk of developing Alzheimer's disease. The MIND diet encourages a plant-forward approach to eating, including more beans, berries, omega-3 fatty acids, vegetables, and whole grains. Vegans can easily enjoy a diet high in omega-3s from sources such as flaxseed, walnuts, and supplements made from sea plants.

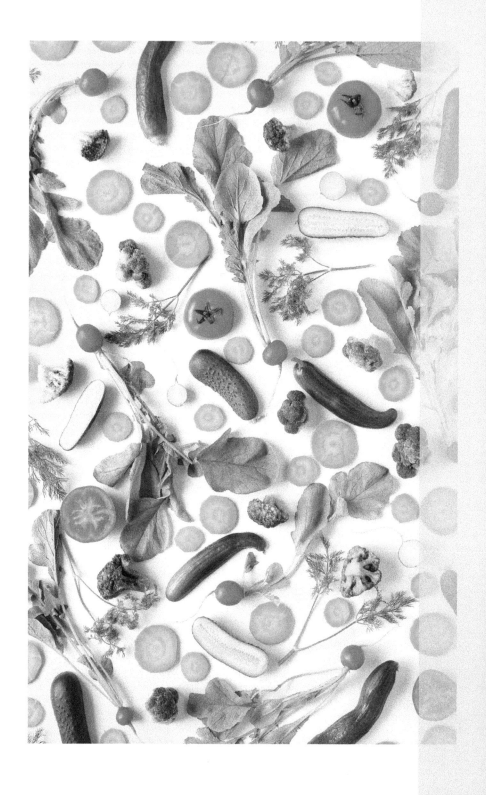

CHAPTER 3

STOCKING A VEGAN KITCHEN

Organizing your kitchen for success is one of the most important things you can do as you transition to a vegan diet. The plant kingdom is so diverse and there are thousands of wonderful vegan foods to eat. You will find it easier to thrive as a vegan when you have a well-stocked kitchen with staples on hand to prepare healthy, delicious food.

Although there are many ways to eat as a vegan, in this chapter, we will dive into some staples and key foods vegans love to have on hand to create the most delicious meals. The foods are organized by type, so you will find it easy to explore and decide what you want to bring into your kitchen.

Pulses (a.k.a. Legumes)

As reliable sources of fiber, iron, and protein, pulses such as beans, lentils, and peas are some of the most nutritious foods on the planet. Pulses are often referred to as "legumes," though technically the term "legume" refers to the entire plant (including leaves and stems), whereas the term "pulse" refers specifically to the edible seed from a legume plant.

The cost of dried or canned pulses is low, and their nutritional value and versatility are high. You will be amazed by the variety of recipes you can prepare with pulses: black bean tacos, five-bean chili, hummus, lentil curry—the options are almost endless.

Dried and canned pulses have similar nutritional values, and each has its pluses and minuses. The canned options often have higher sodium content, are slightly more expensive, and are heavier to carry home. Although dried pulses are cheaper and arguably tastier, they do take a long time to prepare. Fortunately, presoaking or using a pressure cooker makes cooking dried pulses quicker and easier. Whether you choose canned or dried, the following are excellent options to keep in your pantry:

Black beans, also known as turtle beans or *frijoles negros*, are small, dark beans that are popular in Caribbean, Creole, Mexican, South American, and Spanish cuisines. Try these beans as the protein in tacos.

Black-eyed peas are grown around the world, and are particularly important in the cuisine of the American South and in soul food. Hoppin' John, or peas and rice with collard greens, is a traditional soul food, often served on New Year's Day. Hoppin' John is said to bring good luck and is served with corn bread, which symbolizes gold.

Chickpeas, also known as garbanzo beans, are round pulses that are a light golden color and have a mild, slightly nutty flavor. They are eaten around the world, but they are especially famous in popular Middle Eastern dishes such as falafel and hummus, and in the Indian curry dish chana masala.

Lentils offer the advantage that they can be cooked from dried quickly, unlike beans, and yet they are equally nutritious and versatile. There are several varieties of lentils you are likely to find at your local supermarket. Brown or green lentils are the most common. They cook in about 40 minutes and hold their shape quite well. Lentils are at home in an Irish lentil stew, lentil sloppy joes, lentil Bolognese, or a lentil loaf. Red lentils (actually orange) are small and cook in about 10 minutes, yielding a creamy, velvety texture that makes an excellent dhal. Try puy (French) lentils or beluga lentils in salads, as they hold their texture well and look quite pretty.

Soybeans contain more fat than most other beans and are technically not a pulse. That said, they are often shelved with the pulses and have similar health properties, so I list them here. Soybeans are used to make tempeh, tofu, soy curls, and soy milk and are eaten fresh as edamame. Soy foods contain phytoestrogens, which has caused a lot of controversy around their healthfulness. But rest assured, phytoestrogens (plant estrogens) are safe for humans to consume and have a very weak estrogenic effect in the body. Phytoestrogens do not cause increased risk of cancer or feminizing effects in men.

Split peas are green peas that have been peeled and dried. Like many pulses, they are an excellent source of fiber and protein. If you love the smoky, salty flavor of split pea soup, you will be delighted to know you can omit the ham and still achieve that complexity by including smoked paprika in your recipe.

White beans are a general category that includes several varieties, including cannellini, great northern, and navy beans. You may have tasted navy beans as the base in Boston baked beans, a dish featuring creamy, tender beans in a sweet, rich, tangy sauce.

Fruits

Eating a variety of fruits and vegetables is one of the most important things you can do to increase your longevity and decrease your risk for chronic diseases. Researchers in the Global Burden of Disease study found that 2.635 million deaths each year, globally, are attributable to not eating enough fruits and vegetables. They recommended that consuming 600 grams (21 ounces) of fruits and vegetables per day could reduce the risk of heart disease by 31 percent and that for stroke by 19 percent.

Don't be afraid of the natural sugars in fruits. Fruits are naturally high in fiber and water, and you don't need to limit your intake of fruits within a balanced vegan diet. There are many varieties of fruits, including the ones discussed here. Try them all to find your favorites.

Berries are rich in antioxidants and provide more nutrients per calorie than any other fruit. Blueberries, in particular, have a reputation as a superfood, but in fact, all berries deserve that designation. Dr. Michael Greger, founder of NutritionFacts.org and author of the *New York Times* bestseller *How Not to Die*, includes berries in his "daily dozen" list of 12 foods to eat every day.

Citrus fruits, such as grapefruits, lemons, limes, and oranges, are famous for being rich sources of vitamin C. Sour is one of the five elements of flavor, along with sweet, salty, bitter, and umami. Adding a squeeze of lemony sourness to dishes, for example, brings out the other flavors, and the vitamin C will enhance iron adsorption.

Melons have sweet, tender flesh with a high water content. Melons contain many seeds and have a tough outer rind. Some of the most popular varieties are cantaloupe (musk melon), honeydew, and watermelon. Watermelon pairs well with cucumber and mint to make a refreshing summer salad.

Pome fruits, such as apples and pears, ripen in the fall in North America and are eaten raw, as well as used in salads and baking. Try pome fruits paired with autumnal flavors like cinnamon, cloves, and nutmeg.

Stone fruits, or drupes, are soft, sweet fruits that form around a single large pit or stone. Peaches, plums, and nectarines are stone fruits. (Although avocados have a large pit in the center, they are not a stone fruit.) Stone fruits are delicious eaten ripe and juicy, but they also can be added to savory and sweet dishes. Peach pie and plum jam are good examples. Try grilling peaches on the barbecue for a summer treat.

Tropical fruits add a touch of the exotic to desserts, fruit salads, and smoothies. Avocados and coconuts are high-fat tropical fruits that can add creaminess and interest to dishes. Banana, kiwi, mango, papaya, passion fruit, and pineapple are commonly available at the supermarket in the mainland United States and in Canada, although they are not typically grown there. If you like these fruits but find the price too high or the quality too low, try the frozen foods section, where you might find chopped and frozen tropical fruits. Frozen fruits are frozen at their peak of freshness and are as healthy and nutrient-rich as fresh.

Cruciferous Vegetables

Cruciferous vegetables are the most nutrient-dense foods on the planet, meaning they offer the most nutrition per calorie. Cruciferous vegetables are rich in nutrients such as calcium, carotenoids, folate, iron, and vitamins C, E, and K, among others. Following are some common and versatile cruciferous vegetables.

Arugula (also known as rocket) is a slightly bitter salad green with a peppery flavor, originating in the Mediterranean. It is excellent in salads or served raw on top of pizza after it is cooked.

Bok choy is a type of Chinese cabbage, popular worldwide, and typically used in Asian-style dishes. This vegetable has a mild flavor and crunchy texture, and it pairs well with garlic. Try bok choy in a stir-fry or pho.

Broccoli is, famously, disliked by former President George H. W. Bush. "I do not like broccoli," Bush is quoted as saying, "and I haven't liked it since I was a little kid and my mother made me eat it. And I'm president of the United States, and I'm not going to eat any more broccoli!" Bush, it seems, is in the minority, however, in his dislike of this healthy vegetable. Broccoli is the most popular green vegetable by volume of purchases in the United States. Its popularity is understandable; this hearty, mildly sweet vegetable is packed with nutrients such as B vitamins and vitamins A, C, E, and K, iron, magnesium, potassium, and selenium. Broccoli, like other cruciferous vegetables (such as kale and cabbage) also has sulforaphane, a compound that may reduce the risk of cancer and help stabilize blood sugars.

Brussels sprouts look like tiny cabbages and have had a recent resurgence in popularity, having suffered from a reputation for smelling bad (but this is an issue with preparation). Brussels sprouts release a malodorous gas when cooked for a long time, especially when boiled. Try them roasted instead, with garlic, and serve sprinkled with salt and nutritional yeast. Delicious!

Cabbage is a great bargain. Red, green, or savoy cabbage is perfect in soups or salads, and cabbage costs a fraction of the price of other leafy greens. Try pickling cabbage, making a slaw, or preparing cabbage rolls to enjoy the versatility of this delicious winter-hardy vegetable.

Cauliflower is often served as a low-carbohydrate alternative to foods such as rice and pizza crust. Cauliflower wings also make a delicious alternative to chicken wings. When dredged in a coating, baked, then basted with sauce, the resemblance to chicken wings is uncanny—all without the cruelty or cholesterol.

Kale deserves its reputation as one of the world's healthiest foods. This leafy green is a good source of calcium, iron, and vitamins C and K. That said, some people find raw kale hard to digest. Try massaging your kale with a salad dressing and leaving it to rest for an hour, or even overnight, before eating it. You will find it much more tender and ready to enjoy. Kale is also great cooked, and kale chips satisfy that craving for salty, crunchy foods without deep-frying. I love kale sautéed with a drizzle of olive oil and a sprinkle of garlic powder, nutritional yeast, and salt.

Other Vegetables, Plus Tomatoes and Mushrooms

There are so many wonderful varieties of vegetables—this list is certainly not exhaustive. The main idea is that there are no unhealthy vegetables. Set a goal of eating vegetables every day and include a wide variety in your diet.

Aim to fill half your plate with veggies at every meal. This can look like a side salad on every plate, but it can also be a chunky vegetable lasagna, curry, or stir-fry. Or start your meal with a veggie-packed soup (like cream of broccoli made with sunflower seed cream, or minestrone), or try raw veggies and hummus. Starting your meals with a salad or soup and finishing with a piece of fruit will help you feel fuller and meet your nutrient requirements.

ALLIUM FAMILY

The allium family includes onions, leeks, and garlic and provides incredible flavor and health properties. Garlic and onions are consumed almost universally in cuisines around the world to provide flavor and interest to dishes. Garlic also helps reduce blood pressure and cholesterol. Allium vegetables may also help prevent cancer, particularly colorectal cancer. A 2019 study published in the *Asia-Pacific Journal of Clinical Oncology* compared a group of people with colorectal cancer to a group without. The researchers found that those who regularly consumed allium vegetables were 79 percent less likely to have colorectal cancer.

PEPPERS

Peppers range in flavor from sweet to tangy to hot. All peppers are rich in beta-carotene, potassium, and vitamin C. In fact, red bell peppers have more vitamin C than an orange. Bell peppers are mild and sweet and are sold in green, orange, red, and yellow varieties. (They all start out green, then turn red, yellow, or orange as they ripen, depending on the variety.) Peppers are common in fajitas and salads and as a topping for pizza. The banana pepper (commonly served pickled) is a long, thin, mild pepper with yellow or orange skin, somewhat resembling a banana. Try banana peppers on pizza or in a submarine sandwich. Poblano peppers are mild to medium spicy. To prepare poblanos, blacken their tough skins by roasting, then place the peppers in a paper bag to steam and loosen the skins; when cooled, rub off the charred skins. You can serve the peppers stuffed, or use them in place of bell peppers for a slightly spicier kick.

Hotter peppers, including jalapeños and serranos, make good salsa and guacamole ingredients, or pizza toppings for the slightly more adventurous eater. When smoked, jalapeños become chipotle peppers. Thai chiles are much hotter and are commonly found in South Asian cuisine. Habanero and Scotch bonnet peppers are likely the hottest peppers you will find at your local supermarket. These peppers pack a punch and are perfect ingredients for homemade hot sauce.

ROOT VEGETABLES

Root vegetables are some of my favorites to eat. They keep well, are inexpensive, pack loads of nutrients, and have a natural sweetness that makes them family favorites. Try beets, carrots, potatoes, sweet potatoes, and turnips for delicious and simple eating. Beets and carrots are wonderful grated into a summer salad or roasted in winter. Potatoes and sweet potatoes are staples of vegan eating and a wonderful, nutrient-dense option to add fullness to a stew, sheet pan dinner, or power bowl. Try making a delicious vegan mac and cheese sauce using carrots, garlic, onions, potatoes, and sunflower seeds or cashews with nutritional yeast for a delicious and healthy meal without all the saturated fat and cholesterol found in a dairy-based mac and cheese.

SQUASH

Squashes come in two main varieties: winter and summer. Winter squash (including acorn, butternut, pumpkin, and spaghetti squash) are harvested in autumn in North America and have been a dietary staple since Indigenous Peoples began cultivating the land. Beans, corn, and squash are served together in a number of Indigenous cuisines. In fact, the Haudenosaunee, or Iroquois, People began calling these three plants "the Three Sisters" because of how well they grow together in harmony. The plants also complement each other nutritionally in popular dishes such as Three Sisters soup. Winter squash is rich in beta-carotene, fiber, magnesium, potassium, and vitamin C.

Winter squash should be cooked before being eaten. Rather than trying to cut a raw squash, which can be quite tough and sometimes dangerous, try poking a few holes in the squash, then roasting it whole at 375°F for about 45 minutes, or until a knife slides through the squash easily. Remove from the oven, cool slightly, then cut the squash open, remove the seeds, and scoop out the flesh. You can reserve the seeds and roast them, too. The seeds are delicious and crunchy, and packed with protein and healthy fats.

Summer squash include green and yellow zucchini, along with a few other varieties like the gray squash and pattypan squash. The flesh and skin of summer squash are tender and can be eaten raw or cooked. Summer squash have a higher water content than their winter cousins, and a milder flavor.

TOMATOES

Tomatoes are technically fruits, but they certainly don't belong in a fruit salad! They have a flavor profile and culinary use more similar to vegetables, so I've included them in this section. Tomatoes are widely used in many culinary traditions. In summer, fresh tomatoes make wonderful additions to salads and bowls as well as a topping for veggie burgers. If you can't get good tomatoes in winter where you live, choose good-quality, low-sodium canned tomatoes to make tomato-based sauces, soups, stews, and curries. Tomatoes are a rich source of lycopene, which may help prevent some types of cancer and fight heart disease.

MUSHROOMS

Mushrooms are botanically a fungus, not a vegetable, but we use them similarly to vegetables in cooking, and they have a similar nutrient profile: low in calories and rich in micronutrients. Mushrooms are a good source of copper, folate, magnesium, and zinc. Mushrooms can contribute a complex depth of flavor to vegan dishes. Try a blend of lentils, mushrooms, and walnuts as a substitute for ground meat. Dried mushrooms or mushroom powder can be a wonderful flavor addition to soups and sauces.

Nuts and Seeds

Nuts and seeds are a good source of whole food fats, which are an essential part of every diet. Having enough fat helps the body absorb vitamins A, D, E, and K (called fat-soluble vitamins because they are much better absorbed by the body in a meal that contains fat) from foods. Our bodies also benefit from having a good source of heart- and brain-healthy omega-3 fatty acids, which can be found in chia seeds, flaxseed, walnuts, and algae-based supplements. The fat in nuts and seeds comes along with healthy fiber, micronutrients, and protein—as opposed to the fat in vegan margarines and oils, which is not as nutritionally rich. There can be a place for all vegan foods in your diet, but getting most of your fats from whole food sources such as nuts and seeds, instead of from margarines and oils, is a great choice.

Almonds are a good source of calcium, fiber, healthy fats, and protein. Try chopped almonds on top of a bowl or salad for a nutrient boost. Almond butter is a good alternative to peanut butter for those who don't eat peanuts, and it is also a delicious and healthy spread in its own right.

Cashews, with their creamy, rich flavor, are the darlings of the vegan butter, cheese, dessert, and sauce industries. With a slightly sweet flavor, high fat content, and tender texture, cashews can be soaked and blended into creamy dairy alternatives. They make a good snack on their own as well.

Chia seeds originate in Central America, where they, historically, were a staple in the Aztec diet. Chia seeds have a similar nutritional profile to flaxseed. Eating flax and chia seeds regularly may help lower blood pressure and cholesterol. Flax or chia seeds make a great egg substitute when baking. In place of one egg, combine 1 tablespoon chia seeds or ground flax with 3 tablespoons water and let gel for 5 to 10 minutes while you prepare your dry ingredients.

Flaxseed is an excellent bargain. For pennies per tablespoon, you can add this nutritional powerhouse to your morning smoothie or oatmeal, or even stir some into your favorite hearty chilis, sauces, and stews. Flaxseed is rich in protein and healthy fats, including omega-3s, and micronutrients such as copper, magnesium, phosphorus, and thiamine. Flaxseed must be ground for your body to digest them efficiently. You can buy whole flaxseed and grind it yourself, or you can buy ground flax. Once ground, refrigerate flax to prevent oxidization. Ground flaxseed makes an excellent egg substitute in baking and you can also stir it into chili, lentil Bolognese, and other hearty dishes.

Peanuts, though botanically a legume, are similar to nuts and are a very popular food in the United States. In 2020, Americans ate an average of 7.6 pounds of peanuts per person. This amount was a record high, but numbers have been rising steadily each year, mainly due to the consumption of peanut butter. Peanut butter contains 16 grams of fat and 8 grams of protein in a 2-tablespoon (32 g) serving. Try peanut butter on toast, in a sandwich or smoothie, or in a spicy peanut sauce over tofu or noodles.

Pumpkin seeds, like sunflower seeds, are an inexpensive, versatile, and low allergy risk–alternative to nuts. Try pumpkin seeds in bowls, energy balls, granola, salads, and trail mixes. Pumpkin seeds are an excellent source of magnesium, which can help lower blood pressure.

Sunflower seeds make a perfect alternative to cashews in vegan cheeses and sauces. Slightly higher in protein and lower in fat than cashews, they work well with savory flavors. Plus, sunflower seeds are more environmentally friendly, with a lower water footprint than cashews, and they can be grown in the United States, Europe, and in Canada. Another advantage of sunflower seeds is their cost: about one-fourth that of cashews. Sunflower seeds also make a wonderful snack and are school-safe in areas that prohibit peanuts and tree nuts in school lunches because of concerns about allergies.

Walnuts are an excellent source of the omega-3 fatty acid alpha-linolenic acid (ALA). Just 1 ounce (28 grams) of walnuts provides 2.5 grams of ALA. This amount exceeds the daily recommended intake of 1.6 grams for men and 1.1 grams for women. Try walnuts in a delicious vegan pesto with basil, garlic, lemon juice, and nutritional yeast.

Whole Grains

Eating more whole grains may actually extend your life. A study published in 2015 in the *Journal of the American Medical Association: Internal Medicine* reported on findings from two large epidemiological studies following 118,000 Americans. Researchers found that for every daily serving of whole grains (1 ounce/28 grams), participants had a 5 percent reduction in mortality risk and a 9 percent reduction in cardiovascular mortality risk over the period of the study.

Starting your day with oatmeal or overnight oats can be a great way to include more whole grains in your diet. Popcorn makes a delicious whole-grain snack. Protein bowls made with brown rice, buckwheat, farro, millet, or quinoa are another easy option for adding whole grains to your meals. Note that quinoa and buckwheat are pseudocereals rather than grains; however, we eat them as grains and they have similar nutritional advantages—plus, they are naturally gluten-free.

Herbs, Spices, and Condiments

There are so many herbs, spices, and condiments that it is not possible to name them all. I will share a few that I find useful in my pantry to flavor my vegan recipes.

Many spices have anti-inflammatory properties in addition to bringing interesting flavor and depth to foods. Anti-inflammatory spices that are a great addition to a vegan kitchen include ginger and turmeric. Other herbs and spices I always keep on hand are basil, chili powder, cinnamon, cumin, curry powder, garam masala, mint, oregano, pepper (black and white), sage, smoked paprika, and salts (kosher, pink Himalayan, sea salt, and smoked).

Vegan-friendly condiments and sauces you might like to keep stocked in your kitchen include mustards (yellow, Dijon, hot, grainy), vinegars (balsamic, mirin, plum, rice, and wine), soy sauce or tamari, and sriracha.

Vegan Meat Alternatives

Vegan meat alternatives are rapidly growing in variety and popularity. It is now possible to buy vegan burgers, sausages, and "chicken" strips that resemble their meat counterparts in appearance and flavor. The nutritional profiles of these products vary, but they do tend to be high in fat, protein, and sodium.

The fat and sodium content makes them less healthy than other vegan protein options, such as beans, lentils, seitan, tempeh, and tofu. However, these foods do tend to be much lower in saturated fat than the meat products they imitate, and they are cholesterol-free. Vegan meat alternatives also have a much lower greenhouse gas, land, and water footprint. Some vegans chose not to include these foods in their diet for health reasons, but it is very possible to enjoy these products on occasion as part of a balanced diet.

Vegan Dairy Alternatives

One of the most common things vegans hear from non-vegans is "I would go vegan, but I can't give up cheese!" Giving up dairy is getting easier with so many good vegan nondairy options, including vegan butter, cheese, cream cheese, milk, and yogurt. When you're looking to eat healthy as a vegan, aim for options that use more whole foods, like cashews, rather than hydrogenated oils. Fortified nondairy milk is a great choice. (In Canada, nondairy milks are fortified with calcium and vitamins B_{12} and D; in the United States what is added varies.) Enjoy any dairy alternatives that are high in hydrogenated oils, saturated fats, sodium, or added sugars in moderation.

Sweeteners

There are several ways to sweeten a recipe. White and brown sugars are common, but in the United States most white and brown sugars are not vegan because bone char (see page 40) is used in their processing. Agave syrup, coconut sugar, date syrup, maple syrup, and molasses are sweeteners you can use in place of white or brown sugar in recipes (with varying results). Most white and brown sugars manufactured in Canada are vegan. Honey is an animal product and, therefore, is not a vegan sweetener.

When baking, look for vegan recipes that suggest amounts of these substitutes, rather than simply swapping one-to-one with white sugar as they have different properties that may affect the final product.

Other than blackstrap molasses, which is rich in calcium, iron, and other minerals, none of these sweeteners contribute significantly to our nutrition, other than providing energy. WHO recommends keeping our intake of added sugars to 5 to 12 teaspoons per day. All the sweeteners listed here would count toward your added sugar intake. It is a better choice to adjust your palate to enjoy foods with less sugar, enjoy natural sugars in fruits, and/or eat sweet treats less frequently.

READING FOOD LABELS

As a vegan, you will get used to reading nutrition labels to determine whether a product fits your lifestyle. Along with avoiding the obvious like eggs, meat, and milk on the ingredients list, there are a few words you might be less familiar with but that also indicate animal products. Here is a list to watch out for. If you make a mistake, though, don't worry. Being a vegan is not about perfection, but, rather, about making broad changes that are healthy for your body, the animals, and our planet. A slip-up here and there, especially with one of these micro ingredients, won't make much difference for your health, the environment, or the animals.

Albumen: egg white

Bone char: burnt animal bones, often used in the refining process for white and brown sugars in the United States (most Canadian and UK brands of sugar are vegan)

Carmine: also called cochineal or cochineal extract; a red dye made from crushed insects

Casein: a protein found in milk and other dairy products

Gelatin: a protein extracted by boiling animal bones, ligaments, skin, and tendons

Lactose: a sugar found in milk

Lard or tallow: fat extracted from rendering the tissues of pigs (lard) or cows (tallow)

L-cysteine: an amino acid that can be produced synthetically but is often derived from duck or chicken feathers, or even human hair; it is used to prolong the shelf life of some bread products

Shellac: also called confectioner's glaze; a resin secreted by the lac bug, used to coat some candies, chocolates, ice cream cones, and pills

Vitamin D_3: also called cholecalciferol; a common food fortification, usually extracted from sheep's wool (vitamin D_2 is always vegan, and there is a vitamin D_3 made from lichen, available in supplement form, but the fortification form of D_3 is not vegan)

Whey: the high-protein liquid that remains after milk has been curdled and strained to make cheese

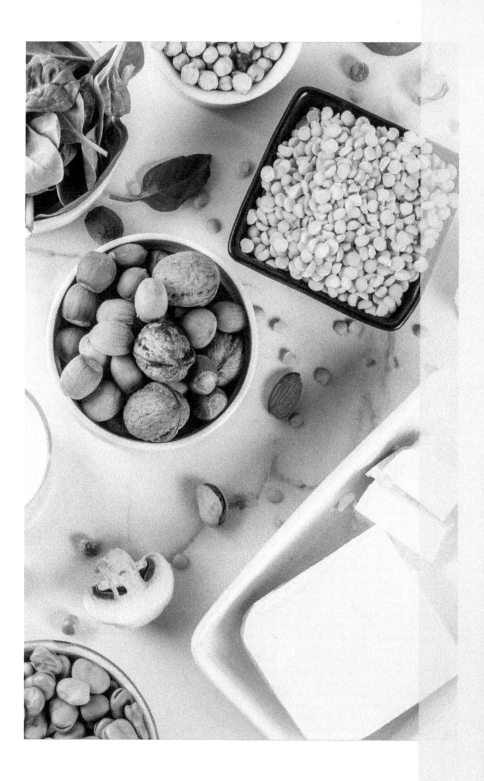

CHAPTER 4

PLANT-BASED PROTEINS

When people think of protein, they often equate it with cheese, eggs, fish, meat, and other animal products and, therefore, assume vegans don't eat enough protein—which is why vegans are often asked, "Where do you get your protein?" The reality is that all whole plant foods contain some protein, and in fact, all protein on Earth originates from plants.

Protein Demystified

Proteins are part of a healthy, balanced diet, and are made up of amino acid building blocks; some of these amino acids are essential (which means that we must get them from food), and some amino acids can be manufactured by our bodies by synthesizing them from other nutrients. We use proteins in our bodies to build bones, muscle, and tissue, and even to make hormones and enzymes. We also can use protein as an energy source. Protein, like carbohydrate, provides four calories of energy per gram. Fat provides nine calories per gram.

The culinary world commonly calls animal- and plant-based foods that are high in protein, "proteins." This is an oversimplification of those foods. Calling foods "proteins" minimizes all the other macronutrients a food may contain. Fish, meat, and poultry contain protein, but they also contain a significant amount of fat, much of which is saturated, or is cholesterol. Plant-based proteins, such as beans, lentils, and seitan, are also good sources of slow-release carbohydrates, whereas tofu and tempeh offer carbohydrates, healthy fats, and proteins in balance. It comes down to what you want served with your protein. For your health, having your protein packaged with fiber and slow-release carbs (as it is in whole plant foods such as lentils) is a much better choice than consuming it with saturated fats and cholesterol, as you would find in a cut of meat.

It's also important to note that protein adds up throughout the day, from all food groups. Whole grains are a good source of protein. One cup of oatmeal cooked with water provides 6 grams of protein, and if you cook it with a cup of soy milk, that's 13 grams of protein. One cup of raw broccoli contains 2.6 grams of protein, and a cup of raspberries has 1.5 grams of protein. A significant amount of protein in our diets comes from foods we don't commonly classify as "proteins."

How Much Protein Do You Need?

Most people who eat a varied plant-based diet have no problem meeting their protein requirements, as long as they get enough calories. For adults (ages 19 to 59 years), the recommended daily protein intake is 0.8 grams of protein per kilo of body weight (1 kilo = 2.2 pounds). On a plant-based diet, it's closer to 1 gram per kilo per day, because most plant proteins don't offer enough of all the essential amino acids in one food, so it is useful to diversify and slightly increase your protein intake. This means that if, for example, you weigh 60 kilos (132 pounds), you need about 60 grams of protein per day. Use the following table as a quick reference to provide an estimate of your daily protein needs.

DAILY PROTEIN NEEDS

BODY WEIGHT IN POUNDS	BODY WEIGHT IN KILOS*	RECOMMENDED DAILY PROTEIN INTAKE IN GRAMS
125	57	57
140	64	64
155	70	70
170	77	77
185	84	84
200	91	91
215	98	98

*All values are rounded to the nearest kilo. Pounds have been calculated using a conversion rate of 2.2 kilos per pound.

Of course, the table represents a general daily recommendation. Every body is different, and some people require more protein. If you're an athlete eating a plant-based diet, you will require 1.1 to 2 grams of protein per kilo of body weight per day, depending on the intensity of your training. Note that 2 grams of protein per kilo of body weight would only be used to support brief periods of intense training, and most athletes find that their needs range between 1.3 grams and 1.5 grams per kilo per day. A 125-pound (57-kilo) athlete would, therefore, require 74 to 86 grams of protein per day. This is attainable eating whole, plant-based foods; however, some athletes do use vegan protein powders for convenience.

It's best to get your protein throughout the day, including sources at each meal. If you are looking to maximize the muscle-building benefit of a workout, have a snack or a meal that includes both carbohydrates and protein within two hours of completing your workout (sooner is better).

Whether you are an athlete or not, meeting your protein needs on a balanced plant-based diet is straightforward and delicious. Eat a variety of protein-rich foods, including beans, lentils, nuts and seeds, and soy products such as tempeh, tofu, and soy milk daily. You may also want to include vegan meat alternatives, such as vegan burgers, sausages, and "chicken" strips, a few times a week.

Protein Quality

Along with paying attention to the quantity of the protein you eat, it is also important to consider the quality of that protein. A healthy vegan diet offers many high-quality protein options to meet your needs. With a little planning and intention, you can easily meet your protein quantity and quality needs and thrive as a vegan.

DIGESTIBILITY

The digestibility of protein refers to its bioavailability, or how much of the protein the body is able to use. Plant proteins tend to have slightly lower digestibility than animal proteins. This lower digestibility is one reason I recommend a higher protein intake for vegans.

Protein digestibility can be measured in several ways, inclu
the protein digestibility corrected amino acid score (PDCAAS).
The PDCAAS for cow's milk is a perfect 1, meaning the protein
in cow's milk is very accessible for the body. Soy's PDCAAS is
also very high at 0.91. Most vegetables and pulses have a score
between 0.70 and 0.78. This score means that if you ate a serving of cow's milk and a serving of lentils that contained the same
amount of protein, your body would be able to use 100 percent of
the protein from the milk and about 70 percent of the protein from
the lentils. Peanuts have a score of 0.52 and wheat has a score
of 0.42.

If you follow a vegan diet, eat a variety of whole foods, and
consume enough calories, then the protein digestibility score is
not something to be concerned about. Research into vegan diets,
such as the EPIC-Oxford and Adventist Health Study-2 studies,
shows that vegans tend to eat enough protein and thrive on a
vegan diet. The digestibility of plant proteins is, however, an argument for prioritizing adequate protein intake. It is one more reason
to include healthy soy in your vegan diet. It is also an argument
against consuming a fruitarian or raw diet; a diet without legumes
and soy will have lower protein digestibility.

ESSENTIAL AMINO ACIDS

Protein is made up of amino acids; they are the building blocks of
proteins. There are 20 amino acids, and nine of those are classified
as essential. Those nine essential amino acids can't be made by
the body, so we must get them from foods. Without all the amino
acids, we can't build muscle and tissue in the body, so it is important to get enough of all of the essential amino acids.

Whole vegan foods contain all nine essential amino acids.
Lysine, however, is a special case, as discussed next.

LYSINE

Lysine is the most common limiting amino acid on a vegan diet,
meaning it is the amino acid most likely to be missing when the
body tries to build tissues, because it only occurs in sufficient

quantities in specific vegan foods. Thankfully, there are many good vegan sources of lysine, and by incorporating these into your diet, you can easily meet your lysine requirements.

Beans, lentils, pumpkin seeds, quinoa, seitan, soy milk, tempeh, and tofu are all good whole food sources of lysine. Meat alternatives and protein powders are also good sources of lysine, if you choose to include them in your diet.

Including a variety of protein-rich foods in your diet each day will ensure that you meet your protein needs, including getting enough of the amino acid lysine. Adequate lysine intake is something most vegans won't need to pay special attention to, but it is a good reminder that eliminating pulses and soy foods can be a dangerous practice on a vegan diet.

COOKING WITH TOFU

Tofu is a great source of the essential amino acid lysine, but it can be tricky to prepare. Here are a few tips.

- Get a tofu press, or press the tofu for 20 minutes between two plates and place a heavy object on top as a weight. Doing so presses out the extra liquid in the tofu and gives it a more pleasant texture. This process also helps the tofu absorb more flavor during cooking.

- After pressing, marinate tofu as you would chicken. Soy sauce mixed with maple syrup, ginger, and garlic makes a wonderful marinade.

- Panfry tofu in a small amount of oil, or crisp it in the oven or in an air fryer.

THE MYTH OF COMPLETE VS. INCOMPLETE PROTEINS

The myth of the incomplete plant protein was started inadvertently in the 1970s by Frances Moore Lappé in her book *Diet for a Small Planet*. Lappé wrote this groundbreaking book to argue that world hunger is not a problem of food scarcity, but, rather, it is a problem of distribution. This book was influential for many people. In fact, I read this book in college and it was one primary reason I initially went vegetarian, starting my path toward veganism.

Although her book's message is an incredibly important one, Lappé also included another message about protein. She wrote that plant proteins don't contain sufficient quantities of all of the essential amino acids, and so we need to combine them in meals; for example, rice and beans or whole-wheat bread and peanut butter. Although these are delicious combinations of vegan foods, and they are good sources of complete proteins, it is not really something we need to be particularly concerned about.

Lappé was correct that the essential amino acids we eat do combine in our bodies to allow us to build muscle, bone, and other tissue. But she was wrong about the need to be concerned about eating complementary proteins (foods that, when combined, contain all nine essential amino acids) at each meal. Although we need to consume all nine essential amino acids, we don't need to eat them together in each meal; we can store amino acids in the body for a while to have ready to use as needed. Just eating a varied diet that contains protein-rich foods will provide all the amino acids we need—in the combinations we need them.

Protein Quantity

Protein is widely distributed across all vegan food groups. The table on the following pages shows the protein content of some sample vegan foods in each food category. Although all whole plant foods contain some protein, the best sources of protein are beans, lentils, meat alternatives, seitan, and soy foods.

PROTEIN IN COMMON VEGAN FOODS

	SERVING SIZE	PROTEIN IN GRAMS* PER SERVING
Legumes and Soy Foods		
Black beans	½ cup cooked	7.5
Chickpeas	½ cup cooked	7
Edamame	3 ounces (85 grams)	9
Kidney beans	½ cup cooked	7.5
Lentils	½ cup cooked	9
Mung beans	½ cup cooked	7
Pinto beans	½ cup cooked	8
Split peas	½ cup cooked	8
Tempeh	3 ounces (85 grams)	17
Tofu	3 ounces (85 grams)	7
Nuts and Seeds		
Almond butter	1.1 ounces (32 grams)/2 tablespoons	7
Chia seeds	1 ounce (28 grams)/3 tablespoons	5
Flaxseed	1 ounce (28 grams)/3 tablespoons	5
Hemp seeds	1 ounce (28 grams)/3 tablespoons	9
Natural peanut butter	1.1 ounces (32 grams)/2 tablespoons	8

*Protein content is rounded to the nearest 0.5 gram. Source: USDA Food Data Central

	SERVING SIZE	PROTEIN IN GRAMS* PER SERVING
Pumpkin seeds	1 ounce (28 grams)/¼ cup	7
Raw almonds	1 ounce (28 grams)/3 tablespoons	6
Raw cashews	1 ounce (28 grams)/3 tablespoons	5
Roasted peanuts	1 ounce (28 grams)/ 3.5 tablespoons	7
Sunflower seeds	1 ounce (28 grams)/ 3.5 tablespoons	7
Walnuts	1 ounce (28 grams)/¼ cup	4
Grains		
Barley, dried	1.75 ounces (50 grams)	6
Brown rice, raw	1.75 ounces (50 grams)	4.5
Buckwheat, dried	1.75 ounces (50 grams)	6.5
Corn tortillas	3 tortillas (1.7 ounces/48 grams)	3
Millet, dried	1.75 ounces (50 grams)	5.5
Oats, dried	1.75 ounces (50 grams)	6
Popcorn, unpopped kernels	1.75 ounces (50 grams)	3.5
Quinoa, dried	1.75 ounces (50 grams)	6.5
Rice, raw (jasmine, white)	1.75 ounces (50 grams)	4
Whole-wheat bread (Dave's Killer Bread)	1 slice (1.5 ounces/42 grams)	4

*Protein content is rounded to the nearest 0.5 gram. Source: USDA Food Data Central

	SERVING SIZE	PROTEIN IN GRAMS* PER SERVING
Vegetables		
Arugula	3 ounces (85 grams)	2
Bell peppers	3 ounces (85 grams)	1
Broccoli	3 ounces (85 grams)	2
Brussels sprouts	3 ounces (85 grams)	3
Carrots	3 ounces (85 grams)	1
Cauliflower	3 ounces (85 grams)	1
Kale	3 ounces (85 grams)	3
Mushrooms	3 ounces (85 grams)	2.5
Spinach	3 ounces (85 grams)	2
Sweet potatoes	3 ounces (85 grams)	1
Fruits		
Apple	1 cup (125 grams)	0.5
Apricot	1 cup (155 grams)	2
Banana	1 cup (150 grams)	1.5
Kiwi	1 cup (180 grams)	2
Mango	1 cup (165 grams)	1.5

*Protein content is rounded to the nearest 0.5 gram. Source: USDA Food Data Central

	SERVING SIZE	PROTEIN IN GRAMS* PER SERVING
Nectarine	1 cup (155 grams)	1.5
Orange	1 cup (180 grams)	1.7
Papaya	1 cup (145 grams)	0.5
Pear	1 cup (125 grams)	0.5
Watermelon	1 cup (154 grams)	1
Meat Alternatives		
Beyond Meat Burger	1 burger (4 ounces/113 grams)	20
Beyond Meat Sausage	1 sausage (2.7 ounces/76 grams)	16
Field Roast Sausage (apple and sage)	1 sausage (3.25 ounces/92 grams)	26
Gardein Chick'n Strips	⅓ pack (2.9 ounces/82 grams)	13
Gardein Meatless Meatballs	3 meatballs (3.2 ounces/90 grams)	15
Impossible Burger	1 burger (4 ounces/113 grams)	19
Lightlife Burger	1 burger (4 ounces/113 grams)	20
Love Seitan Classic Seitan	3.5 ounces (100 grams)	26
Tofurky Sausage	1 sausage (3.4 ounces/99 grams)	24
Yves "The Good Veggie Burger"	1 burger (2.6 ounces/75 grams)	13

*Protein content is rounded to the nearest 0.5 gram. Source: USDA Food Data Central

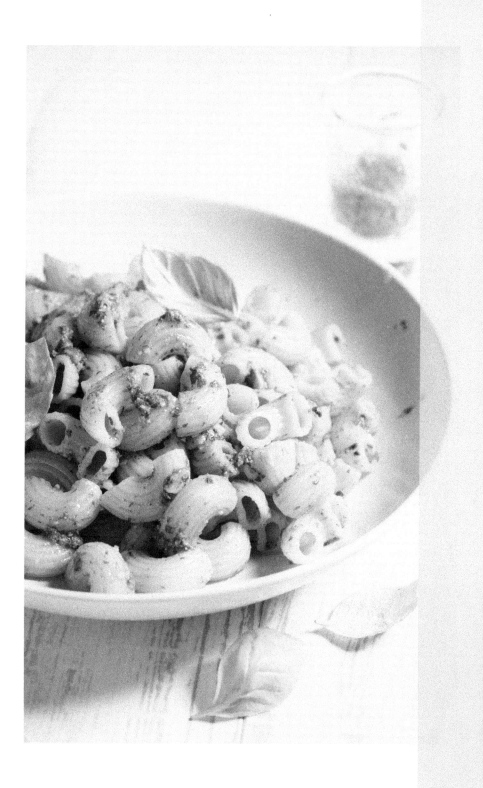

CHAPTER 5

CARBOHYDRATES AND FIBER

Carbohydrates are the sugars and starches found in food. Carbohydrates come mostly from plant foods because plants have the ability to get energy from the sun—something animals cannot do—and, through photosynthesis (the process plants use to turn sunlight into energy), plants produce oxygen and glucose, a type of sugar, a.k.a. carbohydrate. Humans, and many other animals, need carbohydrates for energy, particularly to fuel healthy brain function. On a plant-based diet, carbohydrates are present in all whole foods.

Demystifying Carbohydrates

Unfortunately, despite their importance in providing energy, carbohydrates have a terrible reputation. We live in a society obsessed with protein, where the dominant message in the media is that carbs are bad.

There is, however, a great deal of confusion about what carbs are. Doughnuts and cookies, for example, are often called "carbs." Although doughnuts contain carbohydrates, they also contain a significant amount of fat. A Krispy Kreme chocolate glazed doughnut has 210 calories, and 110 of those calories are from fat. So, a doughnut is not simply a "carb." Generally speaking, the idea of naming any food by its dominant macronutrient is not a very helpful practice when it comes to understanding and building a healthful approach to eating, but if we were to do so, a doughnut would be a "fat," not a "carb."

Given carbohydrates' nasty reputation, many people attempt to limit carbohydrate consumption to very low levels. This limitation can, potentially, cause immediate side effects, like bad breath, brain fog, constipation, fatigue, poor digestion, and overall weakness. Long-term risks of limiting carbs include possible heart disease, increased cancer risk, and osteoporosis. Although the research on low-carbohydrate diets is still emerging, early indications show that, for many, this approach to eating is not a healthy option. Part of the problem with very low–carbohydrate diets is that some people replace the carbohydrates in their diet with fats—often saturated fats and cholesterol. If you want to have greater success improving your health, limit, instead, your intake of added sugars, keep your fiber intake high, and ensure that fat sources are mostly unsaturated (see chapter 6 for more about healthy fats).

Types of Carbohydrates

Not all carbohydrates are created equal. Some carbohydrates are found in whole plant foods, including beans, fruits, grains, nuts, and vegetables. These carbohydrates are delivered to the body in a package of nutrients that includes healthy fats, fiber, and protein. Carbohydrates that are part of foods containing fiber are slowly released into the bloodstream in a sustained and healthy way. Only plants have fiber.

Carbohydrates from added sugars are more processed and have had most or all fiber stripped away. Examples of these types of foods are baked goods, sauces like ketchup and hoisin sauce, and sugar-sweetened beverages. It is best to consume these types of carbohydrate sources as occasional treats and aim to fill your plate most often with carbohydrate-rich foods that are high in fiber. Foods like white bread, white pasta, and white rice have also had some of their nutrients and fiber stripped away. Those foods can still have a place in a healthy vegan diet, but you should choose whole grains more often.

SIMPLE CARBOHYDRATES

Simple carbohydrates can be broken down by the body quickly to be used for fast energy. Sources of simple carbohydrates include fruits, candy, refined sugars, and sugar-sweetened beverages. Simple carbohydrates provide a quick burst of energy, but if you eat them on their own, without fat, fiber, and protein, that burst of energy will be followed by a crash.

Simple carbohydrates can be very useful for athletes looking to fuel endurance activities. Simple carbohydrates also add a delicious sweetness to desserts and drinks. Although these treats can be very enjoyable, consuming them in moderation is encouraged for optimal health.

WHO recommends keeping our intake of free sugars (simple carbohydrates that are not accompanied by fat, fiber, and protein) to 5 to 10 teaspoons per day—though it is important to note that free sugars do not include sugars that occur naturally in fruits and vegetables. The takeaway is that it is healthiest to enjoy added sugars only infrequently, and to savor them when you do have them. If it is tough for you to limit free sugars, try smaller portions, enjoying fruits instead of other desserts, and eat foods rich in simple carbohydrates as part of a meal, to slow the release of their sugar into your bloodstream.

COMPLEX CARBOHYDRATES

Complex carbohydrates are also called polysaccharides and are made up of long chains of sugar molecules strung together, which means it takes longer for the body to break them down than it does to break down simple carbs. Complex carbohydrates include all starches, including white bread, white pasta, and white rice. The healthiest complex carbohydrates, however, are pulses, starchy vegetables, and whole grains, which contain more fiber and, therefore, are digested more slowly.

Grains, such as barley, oats, rice, and wheat, are a type of starchy edible plant. The whole grain is made up of three parts: the bran, the germ, and the endosperm. The bran is the outer layer of the grain. The germ is the seed's embryo, which has the potential to sprout into a new plant. The endosperm is the food supply stored in the grain to give the germ the energy it needs to sprout and grow. Because of this complexity, whole grains are packed with nutrients. The bran is filled with B vitamins, fiber, and minerals. The germ is made up of B vitamins, vitamin E, and healthy fats. The endosperm contains carbohydrates, proteins, and vitamins.

UNREFINED CARBOHYDRATES

Whole unprocessed grains and starchy vegetables are sources of unrefined carbohydrates. Examples include barley, brown rice, buckwheat, bulgur, farro, millet, plantains, popcorn, potatoes, sweet potatoes, teff, whole wheat, and winter squash. The term "unrefined" or "unprocessed" simply means the grains have not been milled and stripped of their bran or germ. Whole fruit and vegetables are also sources of unrefined carbohydrates.

REFINED CARBOHYDRATES

Refined carbohydrates have undergone some type of processing. In contrast to whole grains, refined grains have been milled, so their bran and grain have been removed. Refined grains are popular in manufactured ingredients for a few reasons: They have a longer shelf life than whole grains because they have a lower fat content. The fat in whole grains makes them more unstable and they can go rancid. Refined carbohydrates are also desirable for food manufacturers because they are more palatable and don't challenge eaters with the complex taste and texture of whole grains. Finally, refined grains are easier for food manufacturers to use to create a product that is visually appealing, for example, in pizza crust or sandwich bread.

Sometimes manufacturers add back nutrients to refined carbohydrates to create enriched grains. Pasta is commonly enriched with B vitamins and iron. Breakfast cereals and white breads are also frequently fortified or enriched to replace some of the nutrients lost in processing and to create a more nutrient-rich product. Although these fortified products are often important sources of calcium, folic acid, iron, and zinc, especially for pregnant women and children, it is a good idea to include whole grains in your diet, even if you also eat enriched grains. The enrichment does not completely replace the nutrients found in whole grains (especially the fiber), and sometimes enriched products, particularly cereals, come with added sugars.

Some plants can be refined into sugars and syrups. Sugar beets and sugar cane can be made into molasses, as well as white and brown sugars. Maple sap is processed into maple syrup and agave sap into agave syrup. These sugars and syrups are sources of carbohydrates only and are not a source of protein or fat. Molasses contains micronutrients such as calcium and iron, but most sugars and syrups are refined to the point where they are not a significant source of any micronutrients. These refined sugars provide flavor and sweetness to baking and other recipes, but they do not provide nutrients other than energy.

The Benefits of Unrefined Carbohydrates

You may remember the classic food pyramid from your school days, and so, you are probably somewhat familiar with the general guidelines about what percentage of each macronutrient (carbs, fats, and proteins) to include in your diet. For adults, the United States Department of Agriculture (USDA) recommends consuming 45 to 65 percent of our daily calories from carbohydrates, 10 to 35 percent from protein, and 20 to 35 percent from fat. The USDA also suggests that adults should consume less than 10 percent of total daily calories from saturated fat (see chapter 6 for more about the different kinds of fats). So, carbohydrates should make up the majority of daily calories, and most of those carbohydrates should come from unrefined whole foods.

There are many reasons to include whole food plant-based sources of carbohydrates in your diet. Eating plenty of fruits, nuts and seeds, pulses, vegetables, and whole grains, along with living a healthy lifestyle—for both mental and physical health—will help you achieve the following benefits.

REDUCE HUNGER

Eating a diet rich in whole plant foods naturally means your diet is rich in fiber. Fiber, along with sufficient protein and fats, is an important component of satiety, or the experience of feeling full and satisfied. Of course, satiety is a complex science with both physical and mental components, and can vary from individual to individual. That said, if you believe that a meal will be satiating, you are more likely to leave the meal feeling satisfied.

The importance of satiety is emphasized in many plant-forward diets, many of which share an emphasis on carbohydrate-rich foods. Examples include the volumetrics concept popularized in the book *Volumetrics: Feel Full on Fewer Calories* by Barbara J. Rolls, PhD, a professor at Pennsylvania State University and director of the Laboratory for the Study of Human Ingestive Behavior. Although this is not a vegan book, it does advocate a plant-forward way of eating because the most nutrient-dense but low-calorie foods are plants. The idea behind this way of eating is to fill up on larger portions of high-fiber foods that are low in calories.

Another example of this dietary approach is popularized by Dr. Joel Fuhrman, a former competitive figure skater and author of the bestselling book *Eat to Live*, who encourages a diet focused on consuming foods with the most nutrients per calorie. Fruits, potatoes, vegetables, and whole grains are the basis of this diet—all foods rich in carbohydrates. Finally, Dr. Michael Greger suggests, in his daily dozen approach, to eat foods from several different groups every day, including berries, fruits, grains, and greens. Most of the foods Greger recommends for optimal health are high in carbohydrates.

Although you don't need to follow the specific diets recommended by these experts, the shared emphasis on the hunger-busting power of nutrient-rich carbohydrates is good to note. A large bowl full of an abundant variety of veggies along with some whole grains and beans is likely to be a very satisfying meal.

In my practice, I have seen a wide range of clients with different experiences. Some people seem to be most satisfied by eating a large volume of fiber-rich, low-fat foods. Other people experience immediate satisfaction after such a meal but say that they quickly become hungry again. Fat plays a role in slowing how quickly food moves from your stomach through your digestive system. Some people seem to benefit from slightly smaller portions of plant-based foods, including a moderate amount of fat from health vegan sources, instead of a low-fat diet.

Regardless of whether you choose to include a low or moderate amount of fat in your vegan diet, grounding your meals in unrefined carbohydrates is the healthiest approach to feeling satisfied after you eat. Choose vegetables and fruits with some sources of vegan protein to help you feel full and provide a slow, sustained energy release.

CONTROL BLOOD GLUCOSE AND INSULIN SENSITIVITY

Among other benefits, eating a diet rich in fiber and unrefined carbohydrates can help improve insulin sensitivity. Insulin sensitivity refers to how responsive your body's cells are to insulin, or how much insulin your body needs to produce to maintain healthy blood sugar levels. Insulin resistance is the first step toward developing diabetes, so improving insulin sensitivity may prevent escalation to diabetes, or at least help delay it. People who consistently eat a fiber-rich diet (defined as at least 25 grams of fiber per day for women and 38 grams per day for men) are 20 to 30 percent less likely to develop diabetes. Studies show that an increased intake of fiber can even improve insulin sensitivity. A study published in 2006 in the journal *Diabetes Care* showed that fiber can have a powerful and rapid effect on insulin sensitivity. The study followed 17 overweight or obese German women. Participants who ate bread fortified with 31.2 grams of insoluble fiber (see page 63) each day for just 3 days significantly improved their insulin sensitivity. This is an encouraging example of how quickly health improvements can occur with positive dietary change.

KEEP CHOLESTEROL AND TRIGLYCERIDE LEVELS IN CHECK

Eating a diet rich in fiber and unrefined carbohydrates and low in added sugars can help you keep your cholesterol and triglyceride levels in the healthy range. Keeping these blood lipid levels low will help you reduce your risk of developing diabetes, heart disease, hypertension, and stroke.

Cholesterol is a waxy substance that circulates in your blood. The fatty deposits that build up in the walls of the arteries of people with heart disease are partly made up of cholesterol. However, it is not an inherently bad substance; we need some cholesterol to survive, but our bodies can produce all the cholesterol we need. Usually, when cholesterol levels in the body become too high, it's because of a high intake of saturated fat and cholesterol, which are found, predominantly, in animal products; healthy plant-based diets are naturally low in saturated fats and are cholesterol-free.

Triglycerides, like cholesterol, are blood lipids—fats that circulate in the bloodstream. When we eat, our bodies take any calories we don't use right away and convert them into triglycerides, which then become a stored form of energy that can be used later. If you often eat more calories than you burn, particularly from added sugars, your triglycerides will likely be high. On the other hand, if you eat a diet high in nutrient-dense, lower-calorie foods, such as vegetables, whole grains, and other unprocessed carbohydrates, you are less likely to have extra calories for your body to convert to triglycerides.

Fiber

Fiber is sometimes called "roughage" and is a type of carbohydrate, but unlike other carbohydrates, it does not provide energy through calories. Although the benefits of fiber begin in the gastrointestinal tract, they extend to every part of the body. If you take one piece of advice from this book, it should be to eat enough fiber. It is almost impossible to eat a high-fiber diet that is unhealthy.

There are two types of dietary fiber: soluble and insoluble. *Soluble fiber* swells with water and becomes thick and gel-like. You will have seen this happen if you have ever made oatmeal or soaked psyllium husk, chia seeds, or ground flax in water. Soluble fiber can lower blood glucose and cholesterol levels. *Insoluble fiber* does not absorb water. It is great for increasing stool bulk and preventing constipation.

Every whole plant food contains fiber, and many whole plant foods are sources of both soluble and insoluble fiber. By eating a wide variety of whole plant foods, you will get plenty of fiber without having to specially plan for it.

FIBER FOR GASTROINTESTINAL HEALTH

Having a healthy gut microbiome has so many health advantages. The bacteria in our gut help us digest food, regulate our immune system, and produce some vitamins. A healthy gut can even improve our mental health. The good bacteria in the gut eat fiber. The fiber that our healthy gut microbes eat is called prebiotic fiber. Apples, asparagus, bananas, barley, cocoa, flaxseed, garlic, Jerusalem artichokes, jicama, and oats are all good sources of prebiotic fiber.

Similar to the USDA recommendations already mentioned (see page 60), WHO recommends that 55 to 75 percent of our daily calories come from carbohydrates. This is a good range to support optimal health, assuming that the majority of those carbohydrate calories comes from unrefined foods. It is possible for vegans to thrive on a lower-carbohydrate diet that is rich in vegetables, tofu, nuts, and seeds, and with smaller amounts of fruits and pulses. This can also be a healthy way to eat and is fine as long as fiber and protein needs are being met, and foods are predominately unprocessed.

Whatever ratios of macronutrients are best for you, here is a quick-reference chart of common carbohydrate-rich foods to help you build an eating pattern full of fiber and delicious whole foods.

CARBOHYDRATES AND FIBER IN COMMON VEGAN FOODS

FOOD	SERVING SIZE	CARBOHYDRATES IN GRAMS	FIBER IN GRAMS
Apples	1 medium	25	4.4
Black beans	½ cup cooked	20.5	7.5
Broccoli	1 cup	6	2.4
Brown rice	1 cup cooked	44	3.5
Brussels sprouts	1 cup	8	3.3
Buckwheat	1 cup cooked	33.5	4.5
Cashews	½ cup	19.5	2.2
Hummus	1 tablespoon	4.2	1.4
Lentils	½ cup cooked	20	8
Mangoes	1 cup	25	2.6
Mushrooms	1 cup	2.3	0.7
Oatmeal (unsweetened)	1 cup cooked	28	4
Oranges	1 medium	15	2.1
Plums	1 cup sliced	18.8	2.3
Potatoes	1 medium	37	4.7
Pumpkin seeds	½ cup	17	6
Quinoa	1 cup cooked	36	4.8
Sunflower seeds	½ cup	14	6
Tomatoes	1 medium	3.9	1.2
White pasta	1 cup cooked	43	2.5
White rice	1 cup cooked	46	0.6
Whole-wheat pasta	1 cup cooked	37	6

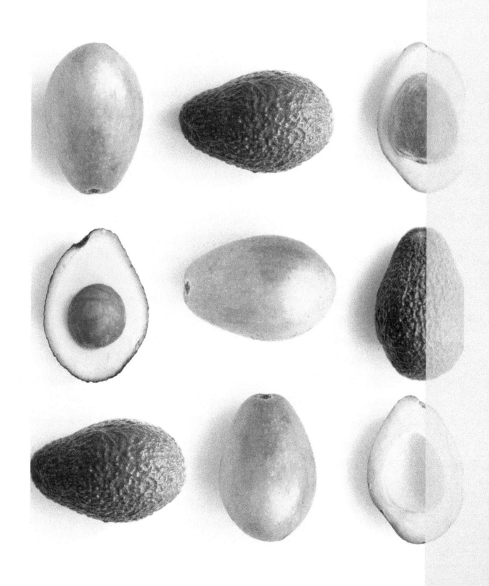

CHAPTER 6

HEALTHY PLANT-BASED FATS

Fats, also called lipids, are made of three fatty acid molecules and a glycerol molecule joined together. The different structures and bonds among these molecules give different fats their unique properties. Our bodies can produce most of the fat we need, but the types of fat our bodies cannot make must come from food. These fats are called essential fatty acids.

Omega-3 fatty acids and omega-6 fatty acids are groups of essential fats that our bodies cannot produce. We can get omega-3 fatty acids from vegan sources such as flaxseed, walnuts, and algae products like spirulina. Omega-6s can be found in nuts, seeds, and vegetable oils.

The Role of Fat in the Diet

Although a diet low in fat can be a healthy way to eat, eliminating fat completely is not. Fat is an essential part of our diet and is required to help us absorb nutrients—vitamins A, D, E, and K are called fat-soluble vitamins because they are absorbed in the body only along with dietary fats. Fats are also a rich source of energy. Protein and carbohydrates both provide four calories of energy per gram, whereas fat provides more than double the amount of energy, at nine calories per gram. Fat also provides texture to sauces and dressings and helps create structure in baked goods.

Omega-3 fatty acids, particularly ALA, must be eaten in our food because our bodies cannot produce it. Omega-3s can help lower blood pressure and reduce the risk of death from cardiovascular disease. On a plant-based diet, ALA can be found in walnuts, flaxseed, and chia seeds.

HOW MUCH FAT SHOULD I EAT?

According to the National Academy of Medicine, the dietary reference intake (DRI) for fat in the United States is 20 to 35 percent of daily calories. So, if you eat 2,000 calories each day, you will need to eat 44 to 77 grams of fat. This is a range, and it applies to a typical daily eating pattern. Don't worry if some meals fall above or below this range; the recommendation applies to your overall eating pattern, not one specific meal or food.

Eating this ratio of fats is fairly easy to accomplish on a healthy vegan diet. Although most vegetables and fruits are naturally low in fat, there are some exceptions, notably avocado, coconut, and olives. Nuts and seeds (and, by extension, nut and seed butters) are also wonderful sources of healthy dietary fats, with the bonus that they also contain fiber, minerals, and protein.

Whole grains are low in fat, though they are not fat-free. One cup of cooked oatmeal, for example, contains 158 calories and 3.2 grams of fat. At 9 calories per gram, that yields 28.8 calories from fat, or about 18 percent of total calories. So, a bowl of oatmeal is just slightly under the recommended range of fat intake, even without the addition of other foods like nut butter. The moral of the story is, when combining a broad range of foods from the various vegan food groups (fruits and vegetables, grains and starches, nuts and seeds, and protein-rich foods) to make delicious and satisfying meals, you will likely meet your dietary fat requirements without difficulty.

Of course, the recommended range of 20 to 35 percent of your daily calories coming from fat is a wide range. It is up to you to decide whether to eat at the upper or lower end of that range. The key is to ensure you eat mostly whole foods from across the food groups.

Diets higher in fat have been implicated in the development of diabetes and heart disease, as well as some cancers. However, in those cases, the fat is often saturated, and the diet is generally of overall poor quality with a low intake of fiber. Consuming fats from whole plant foods at the upper end of the 20 to 35 percent range does not present any increased health risks. That said, if you have a health condition, your health-care provider or dietitian may specifically prescribe a vegan diet that is low in fat.

Types of Fats

There are three main types of fats, called dietary fats, that we get from food: saturated, unsaturated, and trans fats. These categories refer to the types of bonds that connect the carbon atoms in the fatty acid. Saturated fats have only single bonds. Unsaturated fats have at least one double bond: If the fatty acid in an unsaturated fat has one double bond it is monounsaturated. If it has two or more double bonds it is polyunsaturated. The final major category is trans fats. These are unsaturated fats that have been hydrogenated. Hydrogenation is a process that changes the configuration of a double bond, so it behaves more like a single bond.

The chemical structure of fats has a big impact on the way these fats behave in our bodies. In 2017, the American Heart Association recommended replacing saturated fats in the diet with unsaturated fats and/or unrefined carbohydrates. The report underscores that coconut oil, dairy, eggs, meat, and poultry are all sources of saturated fats that contribute to increased risk of cardiovascular disease. The authors of the report also emphasize that trans fats contribute to cardiovascular risk and should be replaced with unsaturated fats. The advisory recommends that the move away from saturated and trans fats be made in the context of an overall shift toward a healthy dietary pattern. For example, the American Heart Association recommends the DASH diet or the Mediterranean diet. Both of these dietary patterns emphasize fruits and vegetables, nuts and seeds, pulses, and whole grains, and deemphasize animal products.

The following sections discuss each type of fat in a little more detail, exploring their role in our diet.

SATURATED FATS

Saturated fats are solid at room temperature because the single bonds between their carbon chains are strong and hard to break. These single bonds make the fatty acids very straight, so they can pack in close together. That feature makes them very stable, but it also gives them their viscous properties, which can thicken your sauces but can also thicken your blood and easily attach to your artery walls.

Saturated fats are predominately found in animal products like dairy, eggs, fish, meat, and poultry. Most plant fats are unsaturated, with the exception of palm and coconut oils, which contain higher levels of saturated fats. Overall, eating a varied and healthy plant-based diet will mean you have a low intake of saturated fats, even if you do occasionally consume palm oil or coconut oil or coconut milk.

WHAT'S THE DEAL WITH COCONUT OIL?

Coconut oil and coconut milk are very popular in vegan cooking, but are they a healthy option? Coconut is much higher in saturated fat than most other plants, so enjoying coconut milk and coconut oil in moderation is wise. Remember, a plant-based diet is generally very low in saturated fat, so unless your doctor has asked you to restrict your saturated fat intake, including coconut fats can be part of a healthy diet.

Because coconut oil is high in saturated fat, it can stand up well to high-heat baking or frying. I have found, however, that olive oil and avocado oil also do a good job at these tasks. Using an air fryer will allow you to get that crispy fried texture with very little (or no) oil.

Canned coconut milk makes delicious curries. Even if you watch your saturated fat intake, there is no reason to buy the "lite" versions of coconut milk, because they are simply watered-down versions of full-fat coconut milk. I suggest buying the full-fat variety of coconut milk and using a smaller portion (e.g., one-fourth can per recipe). You can use almond milk, cashew milk, coconut milk sold as a beverage, or veggie broth to add the rest of the liquid needed in the recipe if it calls for a full can of coconut milk.

UNSATURATED FATS

Unsaturated fats are liquid at room temperature because they have at least one double bond. Double bonds are easier to break, and fatty acids with a double bond will not form in a straight line (they may be V-shaped, for example). This different shape makes it difficult for the fatty acids to pack together tightly, which means unsaturated fats in vegetable oils, like olive and canola (monounsaturated), or sunflower and corn (polyunsaturated), are liquid at room temperature and might not provide the same structure to pastry, or stand up to deep-fat frying the way saturated or trans fats would. That fact is a good thing for your arteries, though, as these unsaturated fats are less likely to adhere to their walls.

Decreasing saturated fat intake on a healthy vegan diet and replacing it with unsaturated fats is easily done. Much of this transition will happen naturally, without you having to think about it, because plant-based foods are naturally low in saturated fats.

HEALTHY REPLACEMENTS

Sometimes, people find it difficult to replace certain elements of their diet. When you're looking to replace poultry, meat, and fish, try protein-rich tofu, tempeh, meat alternatives, or beans and lentils. Replace dairy with vegan milks, yogurts, and nut-based cheeses. Replace the butter in baking with an unsaturated oil, like olive or sunflower. You can often replace half the fat in a cake, muffin, or quick-bread recipe with applesauce and still preserve the quality, texture, and flavor of the baked good.

MONOUNSATURATED FATS

Monounsaturated fats are a type of unsaturated fat that have one double bond. Sources of monounsaturated fats include almonds, avocado, canola oil, flaxseed, hazelnuts, macadamia nuts, olives and olive oil, peanuts and peanut butter, pistachios, pumpkin seeds, and sunflower seeds. Monounsaturated fats are a healthy part of a vegan diet. A 2014 study showed that replacing animal fats with olive oil resulted in a reduction in all causes of mortality, and in cardiovascular disease and stroke.

POLYUNSATURATED FATS

Polyunsaturated fats are a type of unsaturated fat that have more than one double bond. Good sources of polyunsaturated fats include corn and sunflower oils, sunflower seeds, tofu, and walnuts. You will notice that some sources of monounsaturated oils are also sources of polyunsaturated oils. Most plant-based foods contain both types of fat, in varying quantities. There are many trials that demonstrate that replacing saturated fat in the diet with polyunsaturated fat leads to a significant risk reduction in cardiovascular disease.

TRANS FATS

Trans fats are fats that started out as unsaturated, but are treated with a process called hydrogenation. This process shifts the double bond into a trans configuration that is highly stable and very hard to break, behaving similarly to a saturated fat. This innovation was a big success for food manufacturers because it made it possible for vegetable oils to become vegetable shortening and margarine, which can be used in baking, deep-fat frying, and sold as a spread that, similar to butter, is solid at room temperature and spreadable. The problem is that these trans fats were a disaster for our health. Both Canada and the United States have banned commercially produced trans fats. Vegan margarines sold in Canada and the United States are now free of trans fats.

Fat and Muscle Growth

Although we tend to think of protein when we think of building muscle, dietary fat also plays an important role in this process. Fat in your diet helps regulate hormone levels and maintain cellular structure, so muscle tissue can grow. Dietary fat is also important for blood clotting and reducing inflammation, both of which help the body recover from intense training and injury.

Fat-soluble vitamins A, D, E, and K (remember, these are the vitamins your body can only absorb when fat is present) also have a role in helping you grow and maintain muscle. For example, low levels of vitamin D are associated with increased risk of falls and muscle weakness. Vitamin E is important in repairing muscle tears, which is an essential part of building muscle strength, as muscle is built through a process of continually tearing, then repairing to grow stronger.

Having a balanced intake of dietary fats is important for men to maintain testosterone levels as well. Both very low-fat and very high-fat diets can decrease testosterone production. As healthy testosterone levels are vital to muscle building, men who would like to build and maintain lean muscle mass should have a dietary fat intake within the range recommended in the *Dietary Guidelines for Americans* (20 to 35 percent of daily calories).

Healthy Vegan Sources of Fat

Vegan sources of fat are naturally good sources of unsaturated fatty acids and the omega-3 ALA. These dietary fats are optimal for supplying the essential nutrients that fat provides without the potential harm of eating a diet high in saturated fat and cholesterol. Although saturated fat has been identified as a dietary risk factor, and the recommendation to reduce saturated fat and replace it with unsaturated fats and/or unrefined carbohydrates is clear, it is also true that saturated fat has been a bit overvilified.

Much of the problem with saturated fat comes from its abundance within the standard North American diet, which is also full of trans fats and added sugars. It is this overall dietary pattern, combined with a decrease in activity, that is the real problem. No single nutrient on its own, not even saturated fat, can be blamed for the increased rates of chronic disease and obesity.

Another factor to consider regarding saturated fat is that not all foods high in saturated fats are equally risky. For example, 100 grams of panfried bacon (about 6 bacon slices) contains 42 grams of fat, 14 of which are saturated, whereas 100 grams of avocado (about 1 avocado) contains 15 grams of fat, 2 of which are saturated. Although avocado contains saturated fat, it contains much less than bacon, and avocado also contains heart-healthy fiber, which bacon does not. So, we should not avoid foods, like avocado, simply because they contain saturated fat. Avocado—and other whole plant foods that contain saturated fat—can be enjoyed as part of a balanced and healthy vegan diet.

ALMONDS AND ALMOND BUTTER

Almonds are a good source of calcium and protein with a balance of polyunsaturated and monounsaturated fats. Almond butter is a good substitute for peanut butter for anyone allergic to peanuts.

AVOCADO

Avocados are rich in both fat and fiber. They are delicious and versatile and have become very popular for their creamy, satisfying texture. I love to enjoy avocados in guacamole, on toast, or in an avocado pesto sauce. In fact, the first intentionally vegan recipe I ever made was a 15-minute creamy avocado pasta from Angela Liddon's website, *Oh She Glows*. I strongly recommend the pasta.

There is, unfortunately, a cautionary tale associated with avocado. The avocado trade comes at a high cost to the planet. Two small avocados have a CO_2 footprint of 846 grams, according to CarbonFootprint.com. This is about twice the footprint of 1 kilogram of bananas. Water is also a problem; incredibly, each avocado requires 84.5 gallons of water to grow.

Whenever I hear about plant foods that have negative environmental consequences (like avocados, or the water used in drought-stricken California to irrigate almonds), I remind myself that, overall, a plant-based diet has a much lower greenhouse gas and water footprint than a diet that includes animal products. You may choose to limit your avocado consumption for environmental reasons, but if you don't, rest assured that following a diet that includes meat and dairy would use much more water and produce more CO_2.

CHIA SEEDS

Chia seeds are rich in fat, fiber, and protein. Chia seeds are 76 percent polyunsaturated fat, which makes them a perfect candidate to replace saturated fat in our diets to reap the cardiovascular benefits. Chia seeds add texture and interest to overnight oats and make a delicious dessert or snack in chia pudding.

Try this simple chia pudding recipe: Add 2 tablespoons chia seeds to ½ cup plant-based milk and sweeten to taste, if desired. Refrigerate the mixture for a minimum of 2 hours, or overnight, until the texture of the pudding firms up. If you don't like the texture of chia seeds, put your pudding mixture in the blender first, then refrigerate it to set.

FLAXSEED

Like chia seeds, flaxseed is a nutritional marvel, being rich in antioxidants, fiber, omega-3 fatty acids, and protein. It is difficult to imagine a more nutritious food. Plus, flaxseed is versatile and inexpensive—it really is a superfood on a dime.

Ground flaxseed can be used in smoothies, in savory dishes, and in baking as an egg replacement. Some people advise that you should buy your flaxseed whole and grind it yourself. If you are going to do this, a seed mill or coffee grinder works well and makes it an easy job. I find grinding flax to be an unnecessary hassle, so I buy my flaxseed ground. If possible, refrigerate flaxseed, along with all your nuts and seeds, to help prevent them from oxidizing; oxidized seeds will have a sour odor and a bitter taste. Refrigeration is especially important for flaxseed once it is ground, as it oxidizes more quickly.

OLIVES AND OLIVE OIL

Olives and olive oil are rich in monounsaturated fats. Although all oils are characterized as unhealthy by some health professionals in the vegan community, the evidence for that assertion is lacking. A low to moderate amount of vegetable oils, including olive oil, can be part of a healthy vegan diet. When choosing delicious whole food olives, you will gain a very small amount of fiber but also a large amount of salt.

PEANUTS AND PEANUT BUTTER

Although peanuts do contain a significant amount of saturated fat, it is in balance with mono- and polyunsaturated fats, and peanuts still offer a heart-healthy vegan food option.

PUMPKIN SEEDS

Mildly flavored and versatile, pumpkin seeds are rich in protein and healthy fats and are delicious when lightly roasted and used as a crunchy topping for soups or salads. Seeds, including pumpkin seeds and sunflower seeds, generally provide similar nutrition to nuts, but at a fraction of the cost.

SESAME SEEDS AND TAHINI

Sesame seeds are a wonderful source of both fat and calcium. Just 1 tablespoon of tahini (sesame seed paste) offers 6 percent of your daily calcium requirement. Enjoy tahini as a school-safe option to add fat and flavor to children's lunches by using it as a spread on sandwiches or as a dressing or dip. My favorite dressing is lemon tahini: ½ cup tahini blended with ½ cup water, the juice of 1 lemon, 2 minced garlic cloves, and a pinch of salt.

SUNFLOWER SEEDS

These wonderful seeds are rich in healthy fats as well as protein and make a great school-safe snack, roasted or raw. Raw sunflower seeds can be used in place of raw cashews in any savory vegan dip, dressing, or sauce.

WALNUTS

Rich in plant-based omega-3s, walnuts are a must-have in any vegan pantry. Walnuts are a good addition to brownies and energy balls, but are equally at home in savory recipes such as pesto and mushroom-lentil-walnut "meat."

OILS

Some vegans, particularly those who follow a whole food plant-based diet, avoid all oils. The idea is that it is better to get our fat from whole food sources, such as nuts and seeds and avocados, which also contain some fiber, micronutrients, and protein, than from oils where those nutrients have been stripped away through processing. Whole foods do offer nutritional benefits; however, not all oils are unhealthy.

Much of the idea that oils are unhealthy comes from the work of Dr. Caldwell Esselstyn, who saw some incredible transformations in a small group of cardiac patients who followed a whole food plant-based diet. We need to be careful, however, in applying these findings to the general population. All of his patients had advanced heart disease; they were only a small group (fewer than 20); and there was a high drop-out rate from the study. Although this research is worth noting, it is not enough evidence to make recommendations for the general population to avoid oil.

Instead, the weight of research both from epidemiological studies and randomized control trials shows that including plant-based oils as part of a healthy vegan diet can be a heart-healthy strategy. Results from 61,181 women in the Nurses' Health Study (1990 to 2014) and 31,797 men in the Health Professionals Follow-Up Study (1990 to 2014) showed that a higher intake of olive oil decreased cardiovascular risk and decreased inflammation markers.

If you have a health condition and your health-care provider recommends an oil-free diet, that approach may bring about healthy changes for you. Further, if you simply prefer to omit oils and choose only whole plant sources of fat, that is fine. However, if you don't have a diagnosis or doctor's recommendation and are simply looking to optimize your health on a vegan diet, you can safely include a low to moderate amount of oils, such as avocado, grapeseed, olive, and sunflower, which are rich in mono- and/or polyunsaturated fatty acids. Limit or avoid coconut and palm oils because of their high saturated fat content.

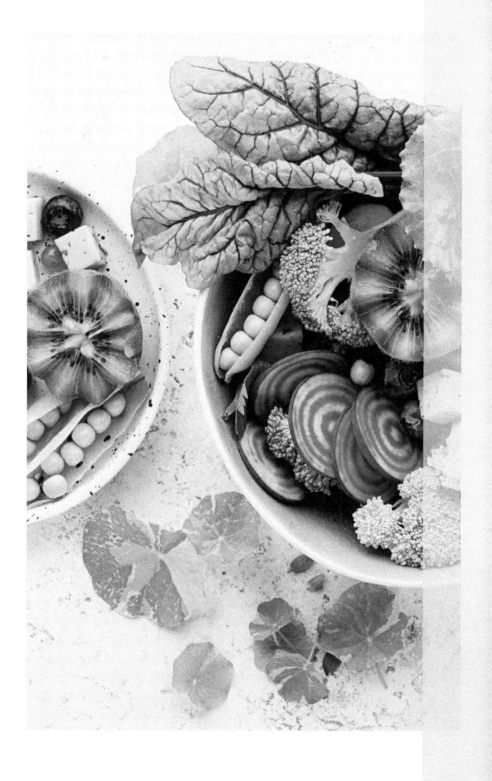

CHAPTER 7

VITAMINS AND MINERALS

As you transition to a vegan lifestyle, you will likely begin to eat more fruit and vegetables and enjoy meals higher in fiber and lower in saturated fat. In this chapter, we'll discuss essential vitamins and minerals and suggested vegan sources for these important nutrients. Some of these nutrients are easily obtained as part of a healthy, balanced vegan diet. Others can be difficult to obtain in a vegan diet without the use of supplements or without paying special attention to adding sources of these nutrients into your routine.

When shopping for supplements, please ask your doctor or dietitian for a recommendation that best meets your needs. Ideally, your supplementation regimen should be informed by your blood work and designed to complement what you eat. When selecting a supplement brand, look for the dosing and formulation that match your health professional's recommendation. The specific brand and characteristics, such as organic or sourced from whole foods, are not likely to make a big difference in the efficacy of your supplements. The supplements that work best are the ones you take regularly, so work out a plan that fits your daily routine and store your supplements somewhere you will remember to take them.

Essential Vitamins and Minerals

The vitamins and minerals discussed here all serve important roles in the body. This section will help you understand which nutrients you may need to supplement, and which can be added to your diet by eating vegan ingredients, such as kelp flakes or nutritional yeast.

VITAMIN B_{12}

Our bodies use vitamin B_{12} to make DNA, and this vitamin also helps keep nerves and blood cells healthy. These functions are very important in the body; without sufficient B_{12} we may develop intense fatigue, depression, and decreased ability to focus.

Unfortunately, there is no whole food plant-based source of vitamin B_{12}—all B_{12} is produced by bacteria, so neither plants nor animals produce it on their own. Meat is a source of B_{12} only because animals come in contact with bacteria through the food they eat and then store the vitamin in their tissues. Farmers also often give their animals B_{12} supplements.

Vitamin B_{12} is found in fortified plant-based milks and nutritional yeast, but people following a plant-based diet should also take a supplement. In my practice, I rarely see B_{12} deficiency among vegans who supplement regularly. That said, it is wise to get your blood work done every couple of years to monitor levels.

Taking B_{12} consistently is much more important than the type of B_{12} you take. You will see some doctors or supplement companies recommending cyanocobalamin, whereas others recommend methylcobalamin. In fact, both varieties are well absorbed by most people. I take a spray, and I find it easier to give a spray to my children, but if a tablet works better for you, that is fine.

The most common supplement options for B_{12} are either a dose of 50 to 100 mcg a day or 1,000 mcg twice a week; just follow the advice and instructions on the supplement package. This may seem like a lot of B_{12}, but these amounts are necessary because your body absorbs less than 1 percent of it.

VITAMIN D

When we think of strong bones and healthy teeth, the first nutrient that comes to mind is often calcium, but we should not forget vitamin D's major role in helping the body absorb that calcium. Vitamin D also helps with cell growth, fights infection, and reduces inflammation.

Although our bodies can synthesize vitamin D from sunshine, the winter sun in cold climates is not strong enough to enable us to do that sufficiently. Everyone who lives in the northern half of the United States or in Canada or Northern Europe would benefit from a vitamin D supplement in winter. In summer months, try to get outside for about 15 minutes of sun exposure each day.

There are very few food sources of vitamin D. Egg yolks, liver, oily fish, and wild mushrooms are among them; however, most people need to rely on fortified foods, sunshine, and/or supplements to meet their vitamin D requirements. In Canada and the United States, look for breakfast cereals, margarine, and plant-based milks fortified with vitamin D. Check the nutrition label to ensure the products you buy are fortified.

There are two types of vitamin D: ergocalciferol (vitamin D_2) and cholecalciferol (vitamin D_3). D_3 is the naturally occurring form of vitamin D that is synthesized in the skin, which is why time spent outside in the sunlight is a great way to boost your vitamin D levels. D_3 is more easily absorbed from fortified foods or supplements, so it is often the form of vitamin D included in supplements. Unfortunately, vitamin D_3 is usually sourced from sheep's wool, so you need to make sure to choose a vegan product that includes either vegan D_3 (sourced from lichen) or vitamin D_2, which is always vegan.

IODINE

Iodine is a trace mineral found in soil. It has an important role in regulating thyroid hormones. Iodine deficiency is a public health risk, so table salt in both Canada and the United States is fortified with iodine. In addition to iodized table salt, sources of iodine in a plant-based diet include sea plants. There is also a variable amount of iodine in some root vegetables, including potatoes. Because it can be difficult to get enough iodine from salt alone, I like to keep a shaker of kelp or dulse (both a form of algae) sprinkles handy to add to foods while I'm cooking. If you prefer, you can take an iodine supplement or select a multivitamin that includes iodine.

IRON

Iron is essential for proper red blood cell function, which transports oxygen from your lungs to the rest of the body. Iron deficiency anemia is the most common nutrient deficiency in the world, and people who menstruate are at higher risk. Menstruating athletes may be even more likely to become anemic. That said, iron deficiency anemia is not more common among vegans and vegetarians than it is among the general population, but it is good to be mindful of your iron consumption because plant-based, non-heme iron is not as easily absorbed as heme iron (iron contained in animal tissues). So, although adults need about 18 mg of iron per day, most people who eat a plant-based diet benefit from more because of this absorption difference. Aim for about 22 mg per day.

It is possible to get all the iron your body needs on a vegan diet. Beans and greens are good sources of iron, as are blackstrap molasses, cashews, dried apricots, lentils, and pumpkin seeds. Vegan burgers and sausages are often fortified with iron.

In addition to enjoying iron-rich foods, there are other ways to enhance your iron absorption. Vitamin C will help you absorb iron, so squeeze some lime juice on your chili or flavor your greens with lemon juice before serving. Cooking in cast-iron pans also increases the iron content of your food. Finally, avoid drinking coffee and black tea with meals because they both contain compounds that reduce iron absorption. Leave at least one hour between a coffee or tea beverage and an iron-rich meal.

CALCIUM

Calcium is the most abundant mineral in your body and helps build and maintain strong bones, and also plays an important role in muscle contraction (including your heart), nervous system function, and stabilizing blood pressure. Health Canada and the National Institutes of Health in the United States both recommend 1,000 mg of calcium per day for adults.

Just one glass of fortified plant-based milk will provide about 300 mg of calcium. To make sure your plant-based milk is fortified, look at the nutrition label. In Canada, most fortified plant-based milks contain 30 percent of your Dietary Reference Intake (DRI) of calcium, 45 percent of vitamin D, and 50 percent of B_{12}. In the United States, fortification varies more widely, so read labels carefully. Most people can meet their calcium requirements easily with one glass of fortified plant milk plus a variety of whole plant foods each day.

If you wish, having two glasses of fortified plant-based milk per day is an easy calcium solution that will provide about two-thirds of your daily calcium requirement. If you choose fortified soy milk, you will also get seven grams of protein per cup. You can add plant milks to your chia pudding, overnight oats, oatmeal, smoothies, soups, and sauces if you don't enjoy drinking them alone. Choose calcium-rich greens such as bok choy, broccoli, collards, kale, and turnip greens, and tofu set with calcium sulfate (check the ingredient list) and tahini to make up the rest.

ZINC

Zinc is essential for tissue building and repair, and also supports the immune system. The good news is, if you eat lots of plant-based protein sources, you will also get zinc. Beans, cashews, chia seeds, chickpeas, fortified breakfast cereals, hemp hearts, lentils, oatmeal, pumpkin seeds, quinoa, tofu, and walnuts are all good sources of zinc.

Dietary Reference Intake for Vitamins

The following table provides general daily recommendations for the most important vitamins. Individual needs may vary, so speak with your health-care provider if you have questions. Please note

AGE	VITAMIN A	VITAMIN B$_{12}$	VITAMIN C	VITAMIN D	
7 to 12 months	500 mcg	0.5 mcg	50 mg	400 IU	
1 to 3 years	300 mcg	0.9 mcg	15 mg	600 IU	
4 to 8 years	400 mcg	1.2 mcg	25 mg	600 IU	
9 to 13 years	600 mcg	1.8 mcg	45 mg	600 IU	
14 to 18 years	900 mcg	2.4 mcg	75 mg	600 IU	
19 to 49 years	900 mcg	2.4 mcg	90 mg	600 IU	
50 to 69 years	900 mcg	2.4 mcg	90 mg	600 IU	
70+ years	900 mcg	2.4 mcg	90 mg	800 IU	

Source: Institute of Medicine, National Academies of Science, Engineering, and Medicine, Dietary Reference Intakes

that this table does not include recommendations for people who are pregnant or breastfeeding.

VITAMIN E	CHOLINE	FOLATE	RIBOFLAVIN	THIAMIN
5 mg	150 mg	80 mcg DFE*	0.4 mg	0.3 mg
6 mg	200 mg	150 mcg DFE	0.5 mg	0.5 mg
7 mg	250 mg	200 mcg DFE	0.6 mg	0.6 mg
11 mg	375 mg	300 mcg DFE	0.9 mg	0.9 mg
15 mg	550 mg (males) 400 mg (females)	400 mcg DFE	1.3 mg (males) 1 mg (females)	1.2 mg (males) 1 mg (females)
15 mg	550 mg (males) 425 mg (females)	400 mcg DFE	1.3 mg (males) 1.1 mg (females)	1.2 mg (males) 1 mg (females)
15 mg	550 mg (males) 425 mg (females)	400 mcg DFE	1.3 mg (males) 1.1 mg (females)	1.2 mg (males) 1.1 mg (females)
15 mg	550 mg (males) 425 mg (females)	400 mcg DFE	1.3 mg (males) 1.1 mg (females)	1.2 mg (males) 1.1 mg (females)

*Folate is listed as mcg DFE, which stands for dietary folate equivalent. It's the amount of folate your body actually absorbs.

Dietary Reference Intake for Minerals

The following table provides general daily recommendations for the most important minerals. Of course, just as with vitamins, individual needs may vary. Use this chart as a general guide and speak with your health-care provider if you have concerns or questions.

AGE	CALCIUM	IODINE	IRON	MAGNESIUM	
7 to 12 months	260 mcg	130 mcg	11 mg	75 mg	
1 to 3 years	700 mg	90 mcg	7 mg	80 mg	
4 to 8 years	1,000 mg	90 mcg	10 mg	130 mg	
9 to 13 years	1,300 mg	120 mcg	8 mg	240 mg	
14 to 18 years	1,300 mg	150 mcg	11 mg	410 mg (males) 360 mg (females)	
19 to 49 years	1,000 mg	150 mcg	8 mg	420 mg (males) 320 mg (females)	
50 to 69 years	1,000 mg	150 mcg	8 mg	420 mg (males) 320 mg (females)	
70+ years	1,200 mg	150 mcg	8 mg	420 mg (males) 320 mg (females)	

Source: Institute of Medicine, National Academies of Science, Engineering, and Medicine, Dietary Reference Intakes

PHOSPHORUS	POTASSIUM	SODIUM	ZINC
275 mg	860 mg	110 mg	3 mg
460 mg	2,000 mg	800 mg	3 mg
500 mg	2,300 mg	1,000 mg	5 mg
1,250 mg	2,500mg (males) 2,300mg (females)	1,200 mg	8 mg
1,250 mg	3,000 mg (males) 2,300 mg (females)	1,500 mg	11 mg (males) 9 mg (females)
700 mg	3,400 mg (males) 2,600 mg (females)	1,500 mg	11 mg (males) 8 mg (females)
700 mg	3,400 mg (males) 2,600 mg (females)	1,500 mg	11 mg (males) 8 mg (females)
700 mg	3,400 mg (males) 2,600 mg (females)	1,500 mg	11 mg (males) 8 mg (females)

TOP 10 TIPS FOR A HEALTHY VEGAN DIET

Tips 1 through 5 are the vegan basics I encourage my clients to follow. Simply doing these things each day will form the foundation of a healthy vegan diet. Work on tips 6 through 10 once you have the basics down and are ready to take your nutrition to the next level.

1. Have at least ONE cup of fortified plant milk each day to help you get your calcium. If you don't like to drink milk, try it in a smoothie or oatmeal.
2. Have at least TWO tablespoons of chia, flax, or hemp seeds each day. Mix it up! These seeds are great sources of protein and healthy fats. They're delicious in overnight oats, stirred into chili, sprinkled on a salad, or blended into a smoothie.
3. Take THREE supplements: B_{12}, vegan vitamin D_3, and algae-sourced omega-3 DHA/EPA.
4. Enjoy foods from all FOUR of the vegan food groups: fruits and veggies; grains and starches; high-protein foods (beans, lentils, meat alternatives, and soy); and nuts and seeds. Include three to four groups at each meal and two to three groups at each snack.
5. Reach for at least FIVE servings of fruits and vegetables each day. Leafy greens and berries are especially good choices. Fresh, frozen raw, and cooked are all wonderful.
6. Don't neglect soy, a complete protein with generous amounts of lysine (an amino acid that is sometimes limited on a plant-based diet). Soy is also a good source of choline—another nutrient that can be challenging to get enough of on a plant-based diet. Edamame, soy milk, tempeh, and tofu are all good sources of soy.
7. Enjoy a mix of both raw and cooked foods. Raw fruits and vegetables are rich in antioxidants, carbohydrate energy, fiber, and vitamins, but they lack sufficient protein and healthy fats. Raw nuts and seeds can help, but raw veganism and fruitarianism

often do not offer enough calories, minerals, and lysine. Include cooked legumes, whole grains, and soy foods with raw vegan foods to ensure a much more complete diet.

8. Eat plenty of whole foods. Whole food plant-based diets are naturally high in fiber and lower in calories than diets that contain animal products, which means you may have to eat larger portions or eat more often to meet your energy and nutrient needs. It is easy to make the mistake of not eating enough when transitioning to a vegan diet, or to rely too heavily on vegan comfort food that is not nutritionally rich. These food choices leave people tired, hungry, and hangry. You will know it is happening if you are unintentionally losing weight. Just start eating more of that delicious vegan food. Emphasize protein and healthy fat-rich foods like nuts and seeds.

9. Include some fortified, minimally processed foods in your diet. Plant-based milks, for example, are often fortified with similar levels of vitamin D and calcium as you would receive from a glass of dairy milk. Nutritional yeast is a tasty topping on pizza, popcorn, and pasta and is often fortified with B vitamins. Many vegan burgers and sausages are fortified with iron, zinc, and vitamin B_{12}. There are many minimally processed foods that are also rich in nutrients and that make wonderful additions to a vegan diet: try canned chickpeas, peanut butter, tempeh, or tofu. Don't let blanket statements about processed foods confuse you. Read the labels and look for foods that are high in fiber and low in added sugars, and that are not deep-fried.

10. Eat an anti-inflammatory diet. Include garlic, ginger, and turmeric along with lots of fresh fruits, herbs, and veggies to help fight inflammation in your body. Try dark chocolate as an anti-inflammatory treat.

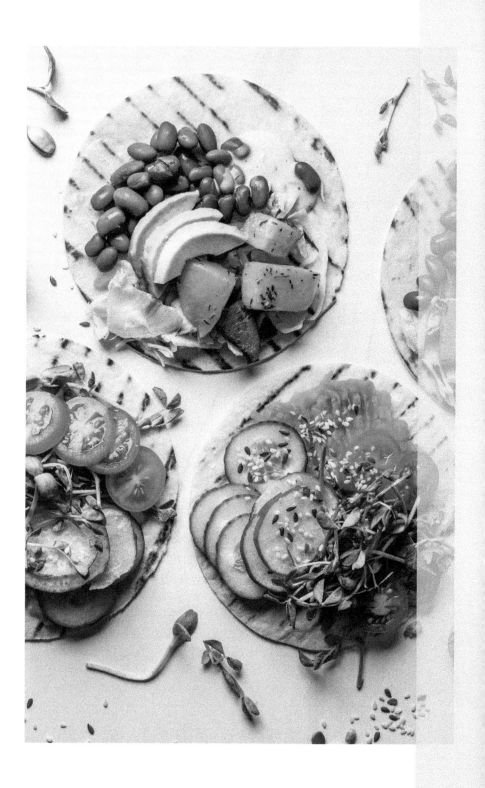

CHAPTER 8

VEGAN FOR EVERY LIFE STAGE

The Academy of Nutrition and Dietetics in the United States has stated that "appropriately planned vegetarian, including vegan, diets are healthful, nutritionally adequate, and may provide health benefits for the prevention and treatment of certain diseases. These diets are appropriate for all stages of the life cycle, including pregnancy, lactation, infancy, childhood, adolescence, older adulthood, and for athletes."

Although it is reassuring to know that a vegan diet is appropriate for all stages of the life cycle, the key to this statement is "appropriately planned." This chapter explores three major phases in the life cycle—childhood, pregnancy, and older adulthood—during which nutritional needs differ from those of a typical adult, and ways to find healthy vegan choices throughout each phase.

Children's Nutritional Needs

A growing number of families are raising their children vegan, either from birth or transitioning to veganism as the children grow. Although raising children with values of compassion for animals and the planet is a wonderful way to parent, it is important to make sure your children's nutrition needs are met. Key nutrients that children need to support healthy growth and development can be found in a vegan diet, mostly through whole foods and with a few supplements. This section will guide you in feeding your children and meeting their nutritional needs. However, you may wish to speak with a vegan dietitian about your children's nutritional needs if you have more questions.

If you're transitioning your children to a plant-based diet, go at a pace that works for you and each child. Speak to them in an age-appropriate way about why you are making these changes for your family. Getting your children's buy-in to the process will make it a lot easier.

FIRST FOODS

It is highly recommended that families raising their children vegan from birth continue breastfeeding or soy formula feeding until at least one year of age. Breastfeeding can be continued to two years and beyond. If you are feeding with formula, speak with your pediatrician about when to stop.

When you are ready to introduce a plant-based milk, fortified pea and soy milks are good options, both being rich in protein and fortified with calcium and vitamin D. However, these milks are low in fat. Children need rich sources of healthy fats in their diet (see the next section), so it is important to ensure they get those fats through other sources, such as nuts and seeds or avocados.

When introducing solid foods at about six months of age (not later), make sure to offer foods from all vegan food groups right from the beginning. Children need diets rich in iron and fat, in particular, so avocados, beans, fortified baby cereals, greens, and nuts and seeds are all examples of great first foods.

FAT

Fat is a key macronutrient for children to support their healthy growth, particularly their brain development. Children 2 to 3 years of age require a total fat intake that represents 30 to 35 percent of calories, and children 4 to 18 years of age need 25 to 35 percent of their calories from fat. It is quite common for young children to lack the necessary fat in their diet. For example, data from the Canadian Community Health Survey in 2004 showed that only 52 percent of children ages 1 to 3 met their needs for dietary fat.

When you feed your family a plant-based diet, your children will naturally get fat from polyunsaturated and monounsaturated sources, such as avocados, nuts and seeds, and vegetable oils. Aim to include a healthy source of vegan fat with every snack and meal. My children particularly love hummus with carrot sticks; apple slices dipped in almond butter; peanut butter and banana smoothies; and avocado toast.

PROTEIN

Protein is essential for growth and development. Although protein is important for your child, children do not have particularly high protein needs. Children between ages 1 and 3 need about 13 grams of protein each day; children ages 4 through 8 need 19 grams; and children between ages 9 and 13 need 34 grams. For teenagers, ages 14 to 18, needs vary by gender: boys need about 52 grams and girls need 46 grams. In most cases, these needs are easily met through a healthy vegan diet.

There are many protein-rich vegan foods that are easy to integrate into your child's diet. For example, beans, lentils, and soy foods ensure a good mix of amino acids. Whole grains, like barley and oats, and grain-like foods, such as quinoa and buckwheat, are also good sources of protein. Nuts and nut butters are also good options, provided your child has no allergies. Nuts and seeds are particularly good choices for young children because they are a good source of protein and healthy fats.

CARBOHYDRATES

A healthy vegan diet is naturally rich in carbohydrates. All four vegan food groups (fruits and vegetables, nuts and seeds, protein-rich foods, and starchy vegetables and grains) are rich in carbohydrates, but fruits and veggies and starchy vegetables and grains are the best sources of this nutrient. As long as your child is getting enough food, they will certainly be getting enough carbohydrates on a healthy vegan diet.

Make sure you offer foods that are high in healthy fats and some protein along with the carbohydrate-rich foods. A healthy vegan diet is naturally high in fiber, which is heart healthy, and also very filling. Be careful that your children, especially infants, toddlers, and preschoolers, don't fill up too much on fiber-rich whole grains and pulses that can't meet all their energy and nutrient needs.

IRON

Iron is essential for the formation of red blood cells. Good sources of iron, such as dark green leafy vegetables (like broccoli, okra, or spring greens); lentils and peas; nuts; pulses (including beans); whole-grain bread and flour, and whole-grain fortified cereals, should be included regularly in a child-friendly vegan diet. Dried fruits, such as apricots, figs, and prunes, are also good choices. By combining an iron-rich food with a vitamin C–rich one, you increase your child's uptake of iron. Try orange segments with fortified breakfast cereal or bell peppers with lentils in a vegetable casserole.

IODINE

The body needs iodine to produce thyroid hormones, which control metabolism and support brain development and bone growth. Infants under six months of age get all the iodine they need from breast milk or formula.

Table salt (not pink Himalayan or sea salt) is fortified with iodine in the United States and Canada. This can be a source of iodine for children ages one and up. Between ¼ and ½ teaspoon of iodized salt per day is enough to meet your child's iodine needs. Children under the age of 12 months should not be given added salt in their diet, as it can be stressful for their developing kidneys.

If you are interested in supplements, you may choose to give your child an iodine supplement to ensure they get the iodine they need. Most children's multivitamins contain iodine.

CALCIUM

Calcium is key for building healthy bones in growing bodies. Humans build about 90 percent of our bone mass before the age of 16, with the remaining 10 percent in the following 10 years. This underscores the importance of ensuring that children have enough calcium in their diets to support bone development. The opportunity to build bone mass closes in young adulthood, and whereas consuming calcium-rich foods later in life can help maintain bone mass, it won't add to it.

One cup of calcium-fortified soy milk will usually provide about one-third of your child's daily calcium needs. Calcium-fortified vegan yogurts are also good choices. Remember, ensuring your child also gets enough vitamin D will help their bodies use the calcium effectively.

Calcium-set tofu, beans, leafy greens, and nuts and seeds are also good sources of calcium. Sesame seeds and tahini are a particularly rich source. Tahini is a good option to include in your child's or teen's diet because it is rich in calcium, healthy fats, and protein, and it is usually school-safe for allergens.

OMEGA-3 FATTY ACIDS

These essential fats are vital for healthy brain development and function. Omega-3 fatty acids are also crucial for eye and heart health. Vegan sources include chia, flax, and hemp seeds, and walnuts. However, because plant foods may not supply your child with all the omega-3 fatty acids they need, consider an algae-based DHA/EPA supplement.

Vegan Nutrition During Pregnancy and Lactation

The following nutrients are important to consider when following a vegan diet during pregnancy and while breastfeeding, as your needs for minerals and vitamins such as iron and folate increase during these times. Make sure to tell your health-care provider that you are following a vegan diet and discuss ways you can meet your dietary needs during this special time.

FOLATE

Folate plays a fundamental role in establishing a healthy pregnancy. It is essential, especially during the first four weeks of pregnancy, for the normal development of the brain, skull, and spine of the fetus. Without enough folate, neural tube defects such as spina bifida may occur. This very early pregnancy development stage occurs before most people realize they are pregnant, so your folate intake should be high if there is even a chance of pregnancy.

People who may become pregnant are advised to consume 400 mcg of folate daily. A healthy and varied vegan diet naturally contains many sources of folate. Beans, beets, flaxseed, leafy greens, lentils, oranges, and peas all contribute to folate levels. However, it is difficult to get 400 mcg of folate from diet alone, so a supplement is recommended for anyone who may become pregnant.

IRON

Iron needs increase in pregnancy as your blood volume increases to support the needs of your growing baby. The iron in plant-based foods is not as easily absorbed as that in meat, so you may find it difficult to get enough iron from food alone. A prenatal vitamin that includes iron will help you meet your requirements. Aim for 30 to 45 mg per day through a combination of supplements and food. Beans and greens are a good source of iron, as are cashews, dried apricots, lentils, and pumpkin seeds. Remember, vitamin C will help you absorb iron, so combine these iron-rich foods with citrus or peppers to round out your meal.

GOOD SOURCES OF IRON ON A VEGAN DIET

FOOD	SERVING SIZE	IRON
Bagel, enriched	1 medium	3.8 mg
Black beans	1 cup cooked	3.6 mg
Black strap molasses	2 tablespoons	7.2 mg
Cashews	¼ cup	2 mg
Kidney beans	1 cup cooked	5.2 mg
Lentils	1 cup cooked	6.6 mg
Peas	1 cup cooked	2.8 mg
Quinoa	1 cup cooked	2.8 mg
Swiss chard	1 cup cooked	4 mg
Tofu	½ cup	6.6 mg
Veggie hot dog, fortified	1 hot dog	3.6 mg

IODINE

In addition to helping regulate hormones, iodine plays a critical role in fetal brain development. If you are accustomed to using Himalayan salt or sea salt, I recommend that you consider using iodized table salt in your cooking during pregnancy. Kelp or dulse sprinkles added when cooking foods can increase iodine content, but these products are very high in iodine, so use them sparingly. Of course, many prenatal supplements include iodine, if you don't want to change your cooking habits.

CALCIUM

While pregnant, you need about 1,000 mg of calcium per day. Just one glass of fortified plant-based milk will provide almost one-third of that requirement. Fortified soy milk is a great option, as it also includes 7 grams of protein per cup. Choose calcium-rich greens such as bok choy, broccoli, collards, kale, and turnip greens, tofu set with calcium sulfate (check the ingredient list), and tahini to make up the rest. Many prenatal vitamins contain calcium; check the label if you are already taking a supplement or when selecting one.

VITAMIN D

Vitamin D plays an essential role in building healthy bones, regulating cell division, and immune function. Vitamin D needs are not increased in pregnancy; however, insufficient vitamin D intake is common in the general population. Make sure your prenatal supplement contains vitamin D. As discussed in chapter 7, vitamin D_2 is always vegan, but vitamin D_3 is often sourced from sheep's wool. Fortunately, there are some vegan D_3 supplements available. If that is a concern for you, look for a vegan prenatal supplement, so you can be confident about the source of the D_3.

VITAMIN B_{12}

Vitamin B_{12} helps prevent preeclampsia, low birth weight, and preterm delivery. Vitamin B_{12} is found in fortified plant-based milks and nutritional yeast, but pregnant vegans should also take a supplement. Most prenatal vitamins will include B_{12}; check that yours does, too.

CHOLINE

Choline is important for your baby's healthy brain development. Although there are plant-based sources of choline (including broccoli, Brussels sprouts, peanut butter, soy milk, and tofu), you may find it difficult to get all 450 mg that are recommended in pregnancy through diet alone. The best approach is to opt for a prenatal vitamin that contains choline or take a separate choline supplement.

OMEGA-3 FATTY ACIDS

Omega-3s, particularly DHA, are important for fetal brain and eye development, starting in the second trimester through the duration of pregnancy. Eating flaxseed and walnuts will help, but an algae-sourced DHA supplement is also a good idea. If you cannot find a prenatal vitamin that includes DHA, you will need to take a separate supplement of at least 200 mg per day while you're trying to conceive and during pregnancy, and at least 300 mg per day when breastfeeding.

Older Adults

Eating a healthy vegan diet can reduce your risk of disease and increase longevity. As the health benefits of plant-based diets become better known, more and more older adults are turning to a vegan diet. That said, calcium, fiber, iron, and vitamins B_{12} and D are especially important as we age, and are worth the extra attention to ensure adequate intake while following a vegan diet.

CALCIUM AND VITAMIN D

Older adults need more calcium and vitamin D to help maintain bone health than when they were younger. To meet these needs, include plenty of plant-based milks, juices, and yogurts fortified with calcium and vitamin D in your daily meals. Calcium-set tofu, dark green vegetables, and nuts and seeds are also good sources of calcium.

IRON

Adults over age 50 are more likely to become iron deficient, particularly people who are older than 85 and living in residential care homes, where the prevalence of anemia may be as high as 63 percent. This deficiency can happen because of low intake or poor absorption of nutrients. People who follow a vegan or vegetarian diet are not more likely than meat eaters to become iron deficient; rather, it is a risk for this age group in general.

Maintaining a good intake of beans and greens will help keep your iron intake high, and including a source of vitamin C in meals will help your body better absorb the iron as you eat it. A lemony lentil soup is a great example of an iron-rich meal that also includes good amounts of vitamin C. An iron supplement may be needed to keep iron levels high. Talk to your health-care provider for help choosing one that is gentle on the stomach.

FIBER

A plant-based diet is naturally rich in fiber, and fiber is an important part of maintaining good bowel, gut, and heart health as we age. Include fruits and vegetables, nuts and seeds, pulses, and whole grains in your diet regularly to keep your intake of both soluble and insoluble fiber high.

VITAMIN B$_{12}$

Like all vegans, senior vegans should supplement B$_{12}$. This recommendation is particularly important for older adults, as seniors tend to have more difficultly absorbing B$_{12}$. One piece of research in Ontario, Canada, found that 43 percent of community-dwelling seniors were B$_{12}$ deficient. With supplementation, however, B$_{12}$ status can improve. Take your B$_{12}$ supplements and get blood work done regularly to ensure you maintain good levels of this important vitamin. If oral supplements are not sufficient, B$_{12}$ injections are an option to discuss with a health-care provider.

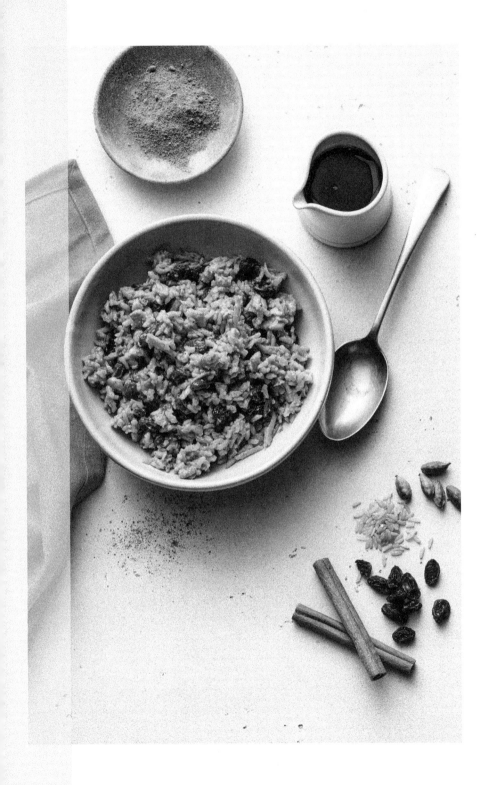

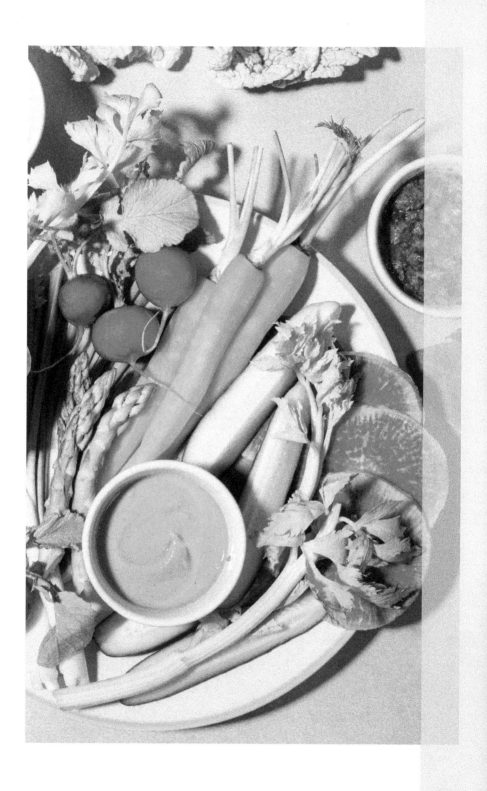

CHAPTER 9

VEGAN ON THE GO: PARTIES, RESTAURANTS, AND TRAVEL

Once eating a vegan diet becomes a habit, it is easy to find vegan choices no matter where you are. With just a little planning and some experience, you will thrive as a vegan in any environment.

At Work

As a healthy vegan, you may find it easier to bring your lunch to work. Check out the facilities available at your office. Do you have access to a kitchenette? Microwave? Refrigerator? If so, it is easy to pack leftovers or simple meals and reheat them at work. As an alternative, consider purchasing a good-quality thermos to bring your hot lunch in. Although I enjoy cold lunches, like chickpea wraps and sandwiches, salads, and power bowls, I also enjoy the comfort of a hot lunch like lentil stew, pasta, or butternut squash soup. So many easy options!

Remember to stock your desk with healthy treats, like dried or fresh fruits, nuts and seeds, and a few small squares of dark chocolate. Finding the snacks that work best for you and keeping them handy will help you feel energized and satisfied throughout the day. Stay hydrated by keeping a large water bottle at your desk. Herbal tea is another great option.

If your job involves a lot of lunches with clients in restaurants, suggest restaurants that you know will have healthy vegan options. See the "Dining Out" section (starting on page 110) for a more detailed exploration of cuisine and restaurant options. When eating out with coworkers or clients, order meals with lots of veggies (aim for half of your plate). Don't be shy to ask for a double portion of veggies or a salad on the side. Consider starting your meal with a big bowl of veggie-rich soup. Choose the whole-grain option where available—for example, a quinoa power bowl instead of a bowl served with white rice.

Parties

Going to vegan parties and celebrating with others who share your values and your love of vegan food can be one of the best parts of following this lifestyle! I certainly recommend you look for vegans in your area who might be hosting meet-ups and potlucks. Join in the fun.

Of course, not every party you'll be invited to will be a vegan party. Celebrating with people who are omnivores and who serve food that contains animal products presents a few challenges. Some vegans find it upsetting to see people eating food that includes animal products. Also, if people at the party know you are vegan, this fact, sometimes, can lead to conversations about veganism that can be confrontational. Of course, these conversations can also be wonderful opportunities to share information and insight about your lifestyle with others, but it is understandable if you find these discussions difficult or intimidating.

Try to find some vegan friends or allies you can rely on at the party to support you, and set clear boundaries if a discussion becomes too personal or triggering. Always have compassion for yourself in this situation; it is understandable when people are curious about your lifestyle, but you do not need to have conversations that make you uncomfortable.

When attending a party, bringing some delicious vegan food to share can be one of the most effective forms of activism. Plus, when you bring something that you will enjoy, you can go knowing there will be something you can eat at the party.

Often, it can be difficult to tell what is vegan just by looking at a table full of food. If you are stuck and not sure what is vegan, don't be shy about asking. That said, there are certain dishes that you can usually count on. A platter of veggies, pita, and hummus, or a bowl of tortilla chips with salsa and guacamole will almost always be vegan.

UNEXPECTED ISSUES

When going vegan, don't be surprised if some issues come up. With a bit of planning and some patience, good boundaries, and communication, you will be able to overcome these common hurdles.

Friends and family don't support me. If those closest to you don't support you, it could be for a variety of reasons. Sometimes a lack of support stems from genuine concern. In this case, responding with a gentle and reassuring approach is usually the best plan. Try to find out what your loved one is concerned about. Are they worried about your health? Perhaps they are concerned that things between you will change as a result of your veganism. Reassure them about your ongoing love for them and the ways you would like your relationship to continue. Also, let them know you have taken the time to learn about the health aspects of veganism and you are making sure to eat a well-balanced vegan diet.

On the other hand, sometimes these concerns stem from cognitive dissonance. People may perceive that your reasons for going vegan (be it for health, the environment, or the animals) are valid reasons, and things they themselves identify with and prioritize. This leads them to the question: Should they also go vegan? If they are not yet ready to go vegan, they may want to discredit your reasons to justify their own inaction. Respond with compassion, but don't get drawn too deeply into discussions with someone who only wants to antagonize you. Draw firm but respectful boundaries and move on to a different topic.

My health-care provider (or caregiver) does not understand a vegan diet. The best way to address questions or doubts from your doctor or other health professional is to share this book with them! Or share other informative documents, such as the *Position of the Academy of Nutrition and Dietetics: Vegetarian Diets* (you'll find it in the list of references for this chapter on page 142). Having the information from an expert source, such as a dietitian, should help allay their concerns.

I crave cheese, junk food, or meat. This is understandable. Making a big change is hard and takes time to get used to. In this case, you might be craving umami flavors, or the combination of salt and fat. Try olives or sun-dried tomatoes, which make great pizza toppings that help replace the salty and fatty flavor of cheese. Meat and dairy substitutes can also help with cravings, especially as you adjust to a plant-based diet.

I need more options. If you find you are getting stuck in a rut and need more vegan options, follow a few vegan influencers on social media (see Resources on page 132). You will find many free recipes and "what I eat in a day" posts that may be inspiring. Pick out a new vegan cookbook at the bookstore or library, or challenge yourself by buy a new type of fruit or vegetable each week and use it in your meals. You can also take a break and let someone else do the cooking for you by choosing a new vegan restaurant to try.

I have low energy. Low energy could mean you are not getting enough calories. Plant-based foods naturally have a lower caloric density than animal products. Are you eating enough? When you transition to a healthy vegan diet, you may need to increase the volume of food you eat. You will know that you are not eating enough calories to meet your energy requirements if you are consistently losing weight.

I'm gassy. It is normal to feel a bit gassy and bloated as you increase the amount of fiber you eat, especially from beans and lentils. Start slowly, increasing your fiber intake with just a few tablespoons of beans or lentils, and increase from there. Drink lots of water, wear comfortable clothing, and stay active to improve digestion. This phase will pass as your body becomes more accustomed to the increased amount of fiber.

Dining Out

Dining out is one of the greatest pleasures in veganism. I have never enjoyed food as much as I have as a vegan. There are many wonderful options, and plant-based cuisine is full of abundance and color. Almost all cuisines naturally include vegan options. Check the suggestions here to guide you when dining at your favorite restaurants.

INDIAN

Because India has a high proportion of vegetarians, the cuisine is full of many wonderful plant-based dishes. Try chana masala, lentil dhal, saag aloo, aloo matar, and vegetable biryani. Indian curries are sometimes made with ghee, which is a clarified butter that is not vegan. Double-check that your favorite Indian restaurant can prepare your meals using only plant-based ingredients.

ITALIAN

Italian food traditionally has a lot of meatless dishes, particularly beans and lentils. Try pasta dishes with tomato-based sauces rich in veggies, lentils, or beans. Vegan restaurants may offer creamy cashew-based sauces as well. Cheese-free pizza is another good option. Try flavorful toppings like mushrooms, olives, nutritional yeast, sun-dried tomatoes, caramelized onions, or roasted red peppers.

JAPANESE

Japanese restaurants offer great vegan options, including an increasing amount of vegan sushi choices. Be sure to ask for no mayo in your sauces, and if you are ordering tempura vegetables, make sure the tempura batter is egg-free. Try agedashi tofu, miso soup, vegan ramen, vegan Japanese curry, and cold soba noodle salad. Delicious! Double-check with your server that these dishes are prepared without fish sauce. In the cases of soups or broths, also check with your server, because some dashi (the broth base for soups) are made with fish flakes.

MEXICAN

There are so many delicious vegan options at your local Mexican restaurant. Try chili sin carne, black bean tacos, rice and beans, nachos with veggie toppings, or veggie burritos. Make sure to ask for no cheese or sour cream. Squeeze some lime juice on top of your food for extra flavor and better iron absorption.

VIETNAMESE

A night out at a Vietnamese restaurant is sure to delight. I especially enjoy fresh vegan spring rolls served with a peanut dipping sauce. Tofu banh mi, garlic bok choy, green papaya salad, and vegan pho are all wonderful options. Many Vietnamese meals are rich in veggies but contain small amounts of meat, fish, and seafood, especially in sauces, so look for vegan-friendly Vietnamese restaurants, or ask your sever to identify which dishes are prepared with ingredients like fish sauce. Fish sauce is also a common ingredient in Thai cooking.

Travel

When you travel, it can be advantageous to book your stay in a place with a kitchenette rather than a simple hotel room, so you can prepare some meals yourself. Restaurant food tends to be higher in salt and fat than food we prepare at home, so this is a great way to stay healthier while traveling. For example, simple breakfasts like oatmeal, avocado toast, or muesli and vegan milk are easy to prepare with limited facilities and will energize you before a big day of sightseeing or business meetings. Consider packing a lunch of hummus and veggie wraps or Greek pasta salad with chickpeas to take along with you.

When looking for the best vegan restaurants in an unfamiliar city, try apps like Happy Cow. After all, enjoying delicious vegan foods is one of the best parts of travel!

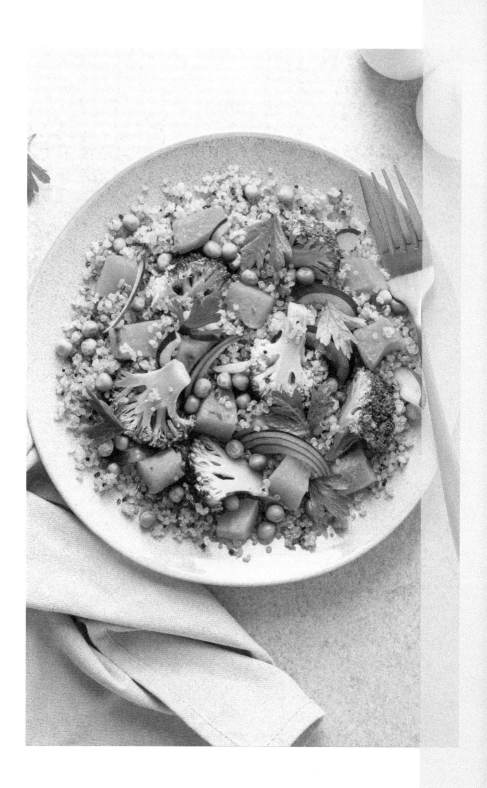

CHAPTER 10

THE VEGAN PLATE AND MENU

If you are new to a vegan diet, this chapter will help you kick-start your vegan lifestyle with ease. Here you'll find simple meals and a week's worth of vegan menu ideas that will keep you healthy and satisfied.

Vegan Staples

There are so many options for vegan meals, of course I cannot list them all here. But the following sample menus feature excellent vegan staples that provide a balance of healthy fats, fiber-rich carbohydrates, and satisfying proteins. Give these meals a try—and also try veganizing your family favorites to create a diet that feels authentically you.

I've provided some portion sizes to serve as a guide. These portions work for me, a moderately active middle-aged female, but there are many factors that play into nutrition requirements. Body size, muscle mass, and age are three of the biggest factors. If you are younger or more active, you might need larger portions. I encourage you to practice intuitive eating. Pay attention to the cues your body gives you and feed it when you are hungry. Remember, staying well hydrated is also an important part of any balanced diet.

STAPLE BREAKFASTS

Here are some excellent breakfast options for healthy vegan eating every day:

Apple-cinnamon buckwheat pancakes: 2 apple-cinnamon pancakes topped with ¼ cup warmed applesauce and 2 tablespoons chopped walnuts

Avocado toast: 1 slice whole-wheat bread and ½ avocado topped with a sprinkle of iodized salt and nutritional yeast or red pepper flakes

Berry smoothie: blend ½ ripe banana, 1 cup blueberries, 1 cup fortified soy milk, 1 tablespoon hemp seeds, and 2 teaspoons peanut butter

Breakfast burrito: 1 flour tortilla stuffed with ¼ cup roasted potatoes, ¼ cup black beans or chopped vegan sausage, and ¼ cup tofu scramble topped with spinach and salsa

Breakfast tacos: 2 corn tortillas stuffed with ¼ cup tofu scramble, ¼ avocado, ¼ cup beans, chili, or chopped vegan sausage, or sautéed mushrooms, topped with cashew or sunflower seed cream

Chocolate–peanut butter smoothie: blend ½ ripe banana, 1 cup fortified soy milk, 1 tablespoon unsweetened cocoa powder, and 1 tablespoon peanut butter

Oatmeal: 1 cup oatmeal made with ½ cup rolled oats, 1 cup fortified soy milk, and 1 tablespoon chia seeds, topped with ½ apple (chopped), ground cinnamon, raisins, and a swirl of 2 teaspoons almond butter

Overnight oats: combine ½ cup rolled oats, ½ cup fortified plant-based milk, 1 teaspoon maple syrup, and 1 teaspoons chia seeds; soak in the refrigerator overnight, then top with berries, 2 teaspoons peanut butter, and unsweetened coconut flakes

Pumpkin waffles: 2 pumpkin waffles drizzled with 1 tablespoon maple syrup and 2 tablespoons chopped pecans

Tofu scramble with a bagel: 3 ounces (85 g) tofu with a pinch each turmeric, black salt (kala namek), dried oregano, dried parsley, and nutritional yeast, served with ½ whole-wheat bagel and 2 tablespoons salsa

Tropical green smoothie: blend ½ ripe banana, 1 cup frozen mango chunks, 2 cups fresh spinach, 1 cup fortified soy milk, and 2 teaspoons tahini

STAPLE LUNCHES AND DINNERS

These staple lunches and dinners will help keep you full and satisfied:

Cabbage soup and tempeh bagel: soup with ½ everything bagel topped with grilled tempeh, hummus, ¼ avocado, arugula, and tomato

Chili and sandwich: sliced tomato and avocado on 2 slices whole-wheat bread, served with 1 cup five-bean chili

Curry: 1 cup chickpea, spinach, and coconut curry served with ¾ cup mixed brown rice and green peas

Kale Caesar salad: topped with roasted chickpea croutons and ¼ vegan Caesar dressing

Large baked potato: topped with roasted broccoli and ½ cup chickpea salad, served with a spinach and tomato side salad with balsamic vinaigrette dressing

Lentil Bolognese: 1½ cups lentil Bolognese prepared with chunky vegetables, served with a side salad

Power bowl: ½ cup quinoa, ½ cup baked tofu, 2 tablespoons hummus, and roasted veggies, drizzled with tahini lemon dressing (see page 118)

Roasted veggie and hummus wraps: enjoy 2 wraps for a full meal

Stir-fry: 1½ cups veggie stir-fry made with tofu, veggies, and brown rice

Tacos: 2 black bean tacos with ¼ cup guacamole and ¼ cup salsa

Tofu pad Thai: 1½ cups tofu pad Thai made with lots of fresh veggies and bean sprouts

Tofu quiche: 1 slice crustless quiche made with chana (chickpea) flour, tofu cheese, and lots of veggies, served with 1 cup roasted butternut squash soup

Veggie burger: served with raw veggies and hummus

STAPLE SNACKS

To hold you over between meals, try some of these vegan snacks:

Apple: with 2 tablespoons peanut butter or almond butter

Chia pudding (see page 76)

Chips and guacamole: 10 to 15 tortilla chips with ¼ cup salsa and ¼ cup guacamole

Chopped veggies: carrots and celery with ⅓ cup hummus

Fruit smoothie: made with soy milk (see Staple Breakfasts, page 114, for a few ideas)

Muesli and yogurt: ⅓ cup muesli and ½ cup vegan yogurt

Rice cakes: enjoy 2, topped with ¼ avocado

Toast: 1 slice whole-wheat toast topped with peanut butter and chia jam

Trail mix: dark chocolate chips, pumpkin seeds, raisins, and unsweetened coconut flakes

Vegan energy or protein balls: 2 balls

STAPLE DESSERTS

When your sweet tooth strikes, turn to these staple vegan desserts:

Almond date bar: 1 bar

Banana n'ice cream: ½ cup

Banana split: 1 ripe banana topped with vegan ice cream, coconut whip, and a sprinkle of chopped nuts

Dark chocolate pieces: ¼ cup

Frozen smoothie pop: 1 pop

Peanut butter cookies: 2 cookies

Sweet potato or black bean brownies: 1 brownie

Vegan cheesecake: 1 slice

Vegan ice cream: ½ cup

Vegan pumpkin pie: 1 slice

STAPLE DRESSINGS AND SAUCES

Jazz up any salad or bowl with these tasty dips, dressings and sauces:

Dips: cashew queso dip, edamame dip, hummus, white bean dip

Dressings:

→ **Maple mustard dressing:** whisk ¾ cup vegetable oil, ½ cup Dijon mustard, ½ cup maple syrup, and ½ cup red wine vinegar until blended

→ **Tahini lemon dressing:** blend 2 parts tahini, 1 part freshly squeezed lemon juice, and 1 part water with 2 garlic cloves, minced; add salt to taste; pairs well with green salads, pita pockets, power bowls

→ **Balsamic vinaigrette:** whisk ¾ cup olive oil, ¼ cup balsamic vinegar, ½ teaspoon iodized salt, and freshly ground black pepper to taste until blended

Pasta sauces: cashew or sunflower cheese sauce; cashew or sunflower Alfredo; vegan pesto made with nutritional yeast instead of cheese; tomato-based sauces using lentils, mushrooms, and chopped walnuts in place of ground beef

Vegan cheese sauce: In a saucepan over medium heat, combine 1 peeled and chopped white or sweet potato, 1 peeled and chopped large carrot, 2 minced garlic cloves, 1 roughly chopped onion, ¼ cup raw sunflower seeds, and 3 cups veggie broth. Simmer for about 15 minutes, until the veggies are soft and the broth is reduced. Blend everything until smooth. Add ½ cup nutritional yeast, ½ teaspoon apple cider vinegar, ¼ teaspoon mustard, a pinch ground turmeric, and ½ teaspoon miso paste (optional). Blend on high speed. Add salt to taste. Variation: Add taco seasoning to create nacho cheese sauce.

Sample Menus for Total Vegan Nutrition

I've designed sample menus for seven days, all of which meet the nutritional needs laid out in this book. If you are preparing to transition to a vegan diet, consider following these menus for the first week, which will give you an opportunity to experience what a balanced vegan diet is like without having to spend too much energy planning it. Keep in mind, the serving sizes here are for reference and, even if one is recommended, fruits and veggies are unlimited; overall, you may need more or less food depending on your activity level, age, body size, and other factors.

MENU DAY 1		
BREAKFAST	1 cup oatmeal made with ½ cup oats, 1 cup fortified soy milk, and 1 tablespoon chia seeds topped with ½ apple (chopped), ground cinnamon, raisins, and 2 teaspoons almond butter	**PER SERVING:** **Calories:** 415 **Total fat:** 15.5g **Sodium:** 115.9mg **Carbohydrates:** 56.9g **Fiber:** 13.8g **Sugars:** 17.3g **Protein:** 17.5g
LUNCH	Avocado and tomato sandwich on 2 slices whole-wheat bread, served with 1 cup five-bean chili	**PER SERVING:** **Calories:** 449 **Total fat:** 14g **Sodium:** 802mg **Carbohydrates:** 65.5g **Fiber:** 18.2g **Sugars:** 10.9g **Protein:** 19.5g
SNACK	Apple with 2 tablespoons peanut butter	**PER SERVING:** **Calories:** 283 **Total fat:** 16.2g **Sodium:** 3.7mg **Carbohydrates:** 31.9g **Fiber:** 7.1g **Sugars:** 20.5g **Protein:** 8.3g
DINNER	1 large baked potato topped with roasted broccoli and ½ cup chickpea salad, plus a spinach and tomato side salad with 2 tablespoons balsamic vinaigrette (see page 118)	**PER SERVING:** **Calories:** 603 **Total fat:** 21.2g **Sodium:** 705mg **Carbohydrates:** 94.7g **Fiber:** 14.5g **Sugars:** 16.6g **Protein:** 16.8g

Daily Total: Calories: 1,750; Total fat: 66.9g; Sodium: 1,626.6mg; Carbohydrates: 249g; Fiber: 53.6; Sugars: 65.3g; Protein: 62.1g

MENU DAY 2		
BREAKFAST	Chocolate–peanut butter smoothie made with 2 cups chopped kale, 1 cup fortified soy milk, ½ ripe banana, 1 tablespoon unsweetened cocoa powder, and 1 tablespoon peanut butter	**PER SERVING:** **Calories:** 253 **Total fat:** 11g **Sodium:** 126mg **Carbohydrates:** 28g **Fiber:** 5g **Sugars:** 12g **Protein:** 13g
LUNCH	Veggie stir-fry made with 3 ounces (85 g) tofu, 1½ cups mixed veggies, ¾ cup brown rice	**PER SERVING:** **Calories:** 398 **Total fat:** 15g **Sodium:** 986mg **Carbohydrates:** 53g **Fiber:** 7g **Sugars:** 4g **Protein:** 14g
SNACK	½ cup carrot sticks, ½ cup celery sticks, ⅓ cup hummus	**PER SERVING:** **Calories:** 219 **Total fat:** 13g **Sodium:** 427mg **Carbohydrates:** 18g **Fiber:** 8g **Sugars:** 7g **Protein:** 6g
DINNER	Power bowl made with ½ cup quinoa, 3 ounces (85 g) tofu, baked, 2 tablespoons hummus, and roasted veggies, drizzled with 2 tablespoons tahini lemon dressing (see page 118)	**PER SERVING:** **Calories:** 526 **Total fat:** 23g **Sodium:** 247mg **Carbohydrates:** 54g **Fiber:** 36g **Sugars:** 1g **Protein:** 19g

Daily Total: Calories: 1,396; Total fat: 62g; Sodium: 1,786mg; Carbohydrates: 163g; Fiber: 56g; Sugars: 24g; Protein: 52g

MENU DAY 3		
BREAKFAST	2 apple-cinnamon pancakes topped with ¼ cup warmed applesauce and 2 tablespoons chopped walnuts	**PER SERVING:** **Calories:** 168 **Total fat:** 5g **Sodium:** 340mg **Carbohydrates:** 27g **Fiber:** 5g **Sugars:** 8g **Protein:** 3g
LUNCH	Veggie burger on a whole-wheat bun topped with lettuce, tomato, and pickle, served with chopped red bell pepper and cucumber with edamame dip	**PER SERVING:** **Calories:** 516 **Total fat:** 24g **Sodium:** 1,474mg **Carbohydrates:** 55g **Fiber:** 11g **Sugars:** 11g **Protein:** 26g
SNACK	10 tortilla chips with ¼ cup salsa and ¼ cup guacamole	**PER SERVING:** **Calories:** 280 **Total fat:** 17g **Sodium:** 375mg **Carbohydrates:** 26g **Fiber:** 4g **Sugars:** 2g **Protein:** 5g
DINNER	Kale Caesar salad with ½ cup roasted chickpeas and ¼ vegan Caesar dressing	**PER SERVING:** **Calories:** 610 **Total fat:** 35g **Sodium:** 818mg **Carbohydrates:** 58g **Fiber:** 14g **Sugars:** 6g **Protein:** 20g

Daily Total: Calories: 1,574; Total fat: 81g; Sodium: 3,007mg; Carbohydrates: 166g; Fiber: 34g; Sugars: 27g; Protein: 54g

MENU DAY 4		
BREAKFAST	Tropical green smoothie made with 2 cups fresh spinach, 1 cup frozen mango chunks, 1 cup fortified soy milk, ½ ripe banana, and 2 teaspoons tahini	**PER SERVING:** **Calories:** 290 **Total fat:** 10g **Sodium:** 118mg **Carbohydrates:** 43g **Fiber:** 7g **Sugars:** 27g **Protein:** 13g
LUNCH	1½ cups lentil Bolognese prepared with chunky vegetables and served with a side salad	**PER SERVING:** **Calories:** 394 **Total fat:** 16g **Sodium:** 1,346mg **Carbohydrates:** 52g **Fiber:** 12g **Sugars:** 14g **Protein:** 14g
SNACK	½ cup chia pudding (see page 76)	**PER SERVING:** **Calories:** 143 **Total fat:** 9g **Sodium:** 0mg **Carbohydrates:** 2g **Fiber:** 11g **Sugars:** 0g **Protein:** 5g
DINNER	1 cup tofu pad Thai made with lots of fresh veggies and bean sprouts	**PER SERVING:** **Calories:** 600 **Total fat:** 7g **Sodium:** 840mg **Carbohydrates:** 114g **Fiber:** 3g **Sugars:** 23g **Protein:** 18g

Daily Total: Calories: 1,427; Total fat: 42g; Sodium: 2,304mg; Carbohydrates: 211g; Fiber: 33g; Sugars: 64g; Protein: 50g

MENU DAY 5

BREAKFAST	Tofu scramble made with 3 ounces (85 g) tofu, pinch each ground turmeric, black salt (kala namek), dried oregano, dried parsley, and nutritional yeast, served with ½ whole-wheat bagel and 2 tablespoons salsa	**PER SERVING:** **Calories:** 313 **Total fat:** 9g **Sodium:** 375mg **Carbohydrates:** 31g **Fiber:** 8g **Sugars:** 4g **Protein:** 31g
LUNCH	1 cup chickpea, spinach, and coconut curry with ¾ cup mixed brown rice and green peas	**PER SERVING:** **Calories:** 426 **Total fat:** 10g **Sodium:** 819mg **Carbohydrates:** 69g **Fiber:** 22g **Sugars:** 5g **Protein:** 15g
SNACK	2 vegan energy balls	**PER SERVING:** **Calories:** 210 **Total fat:** 8g **Sodium:** 0mg **Carbohydrates:** 21g **Fiber:** 3g **Sugars:** 12g **Protein:** 12g
DINNER	2 black bean tacos, with ¼ cup guacamole and ¼ cup salsa	**PER SERVING:** **Calories:** 491 **Total fat:** 12g **Sodium:** 946mg **Carbohydrates:** 77g **Fiber:** 19g **Sugars:** 2g **Protein:** 21g

Daily Total: Calories: 1,440; Total fat: 39g; Sodium: 2,140mg; Carbohydrates: 198g; Fiber: 53g; Sugars: 23g; Protein: 79g

MENU DAY 6		
BREAKFAST	2 pumpkin waffles drizzled with 1 tablespoon maple syrup and 2 tablespoons chopped pecans	**PER SERVING:** **Calories:** 447 **Total fat:** 22g **Sodium:** 411mg **Carbohydrates:** 53g **Fiber:** 7g **Sugars:** 23g **Protein:** 10g
LUNCH	1 cup hot-and-sour cabbage soup and ½ everything bagel, with 1½ ounces grilled tempeh, hummus, ¼ avocado, arugula, and tomato	**PER SERVING:** **Calories:** 506 **Total fat:** 15g **Sodium:** 3,625mg **Carbohydrates:** 71g **Fiber:** 17g **Sugars:** 8g **Protein:** 24g
SNACK	3 cups air-popped popcorn	**PER SERVING:** **Calories:** 48 **Total fat:** 1g **Sodium:** 0mg **Carbohydrates:** 12g **Fiber:** 2g **Sugars:** 0g **Protein:** 2g
DINNER	1 cup vegan mushroom and pea risotto	**PER SERVING:** **Calories:** 472 **Total fat:** 11g **Sodium:** 1,895mg **Carbohydrates:** 75g **Fiber:** 7g **Sugars:** 6g **Protein:** 17g

Daily Total: Calories: 1,473; Total fat: 49g; Sodium: 5,931mg; Carbohydrates: 211g; Fiber: 30g; Sugars: 37g; Protein: 53g

MENU DAY 7		
BREAKFAST	Overnight oats (see page 115)	**PER SERVING:** **Calories:** 489 **Total fat:** 20g **Sodium:** 64mg **Carbohydrates:** 71g **Fiber:** 14g **Sugars:** 24g **Protein:** 13g
LUNCH	Roasted veggie and hummus wrap	**PER SERVING:** **Calories:** 490 **Total fat:** 15g **Sodium:** 1,050mg **Carbohydrates:** 76g **Fiber:** 9g **Sugars:** 8g **Protein:** 15g
SNACK	½ cup banana n'ice cream	**PER SERVING:** **Calories:** 105 **Total fat:** 0g **Sodium:** 1mg **Carbohydrates:** 27g **Fiber:** 3g **Sugars:** 14g **Protein:** 1g
DINNER	1 slice crustless quiche made with chana flour, tofu cheese, and lots of veggies, with 1 cup roasted butternut squash soup	**PER SERVING:** **Calories:** 643 **Total fat:** 28g **Sodium:** 789mg **Carbohydrates:** 67g **Fiber:** 11g **Sugars:** 8g **Protein:** 22g

Daily Total: Calories: 1,727; Total fat: 63g; Sodium: 1,904mg; Carbohydrates: 241g; Fiber: 37g; Sugars: 54g; Protein: 51g

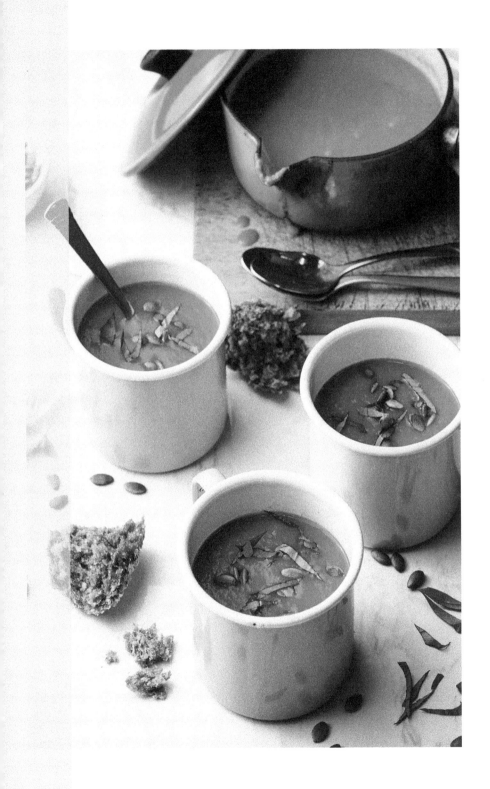

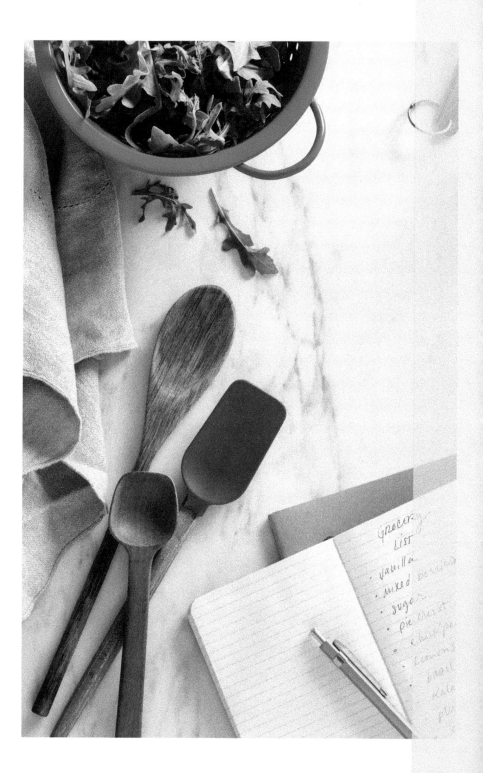

Grocery
List

· Vanilla
· mixed berries
· sugar
· pie crust
· chickpeas
· lemons
· basil
· kale
· pineapple

RESOURCES

COOKBOOKS

Forks Over Knives—The Cookbook by Del Sroufe with Isa Chandra Moskowitz (The Experiment, 2012)

From the same people who brought you the documentary of the same name, this cookbook is the bible of whole food plant-based recipes. If you are looking for whole food plant-based options with no oil, this is an excellent resource.

Fuss-Free Vegan: 101 Everyday Comfort Food Favorites, Veganized by Sam Turnbull (Appetite by Random House, 2017)

These recipes work every time! Sam really knows comfort food, and if you are missing any classics from your pre-vegan days, these recipes will hit the spot.

Oh She Glows Every Day by Angela Liddon (Avery, 2016)

Angela's recipes are healthy, delicious, and beautiful. I love this particular collection because they are simple enough for every day but special enough for an occasion.

Vegan Richa's Indian Kitchen by Richa Hingle (Vegan Heritage Press, 2015)

Indian cuisine has so much to offer vegans as many recipes are naturally plant-based. You will love all the ways to use lentils and beans, and the spices will make your food naturally flavorful. Richa takes you through each recipe and technique, so even someone new to Indian cooking will get great results.

Vegetable Kingdom: The Abundant World of Vegan Recipes by Bryant Terry (Ten Speed Press, 2020)

This beautiful cookbook will teach you the fundamentals of vegan cooking, focusing on whole foods.

HELPFUL BOOKS FOR VEGANS

The Alzheimer's Solution: A Breakthrough Program to Prevent and Reverse the Symptoms of Cognitive Decline at Every Age by Dr. Dean Sherzai and Dr. Ayesha Sherzai (HarperOne, 2019)

Learning how to reduce your risk of developing dementia is one of the most important things you can do for your health. This book offers practical solutions with a focus on plant-based nutrition.

The China Study: The Most Comprehensive Study of Nutrition Ever Conducted and the Startling Implications for Diet, Weight Loss, and Long-Term Health, by Dr. T. Colin Campbell and Dr. Thomas M. Campbell II (BenBella Books, 2016)

This study had a powerful impact on the nutrition world. This fascinating and easy-to-understand account of the research will inspire you to eat more plants and help you understand why it is important to do so.

Dr. Neal Barnard's Program for Reversing Diabetes: The Scientifically Proven System for Reversing Diabetes without Drugs by Dr. Neal Barnard (Rodale Books, 2018)

If you or someone you love has diabetes, this program can help you control your blood sugars and reduce your risk of complications naturally with healthy foods.

Eating Animals by Jonathan Safran Foer (Back Bay Books, 2010)

A hard-hitting, honest account of the process of how animal products end up on our plates.

Even Vegans Die: A Practical Guide to Caregiving, Acceptance, and Protecting Your Legacy of Compassion by Carol J. Adams, Patti Breitman, and Virginia Messina (Lantern Books, 2017)

This beautiful book takes a compassionate approach to preparing for end of life and acknowledging that although a plant-based diet does have health benefits, there are no guarantees of health with any diet.

Fiber Fueled: The Plant-Based Gut Health Program for Losing Weight, Restoring Your Health, and Optimizing Your Microbiome by Dr. Will Bulsiewicz (Avery, 2020)

This book makes fiber sexy—not an easy task—but Dr. B is getting everyone's attention for this often-overlooked nutrient that is actually one of the most important keys to health. Following the protocol outlined in this book will revolutionize your health.

How Not to Die by Dr. Michael Greger with Gene Stone (Flatiron Books, 2015)

This comprehensive book discusses all the most common diseases experienced by North Americans, and how to prevent them using simple diet and lifestyle habits.

How Not to Diet by Dr. Michael Greger (Flatiron Books, 2019)

In this book, Michael Greger discusses the science of achieving and maintaining a healthy weight.

Why We Love Dogs, Eat Pigs, and Wear Cows: An Introduction to Carnism by Dr. Melanie Joy (Red Wheel, 2020)

An excellent book that challenges many of our societal norms about animals.

WEBSITES

Forks Over Knives
forksoverknives.com
This site is packed with tools, recipes, guides, and inspirational stories.

Mercy for Animals
mercyforanimals.org
Want to know more about the conditions of animals in animal agriculture? This site has the information and ways to advocate for animals.

Our Hen House
ourhenhouse.org
This wonderful podcast has been changing the world for animals with weekly episodes since 2017.

Physicians Committee for Responsible Medicine

pcrm.org

Looking for the science behind a plant-based diet? This site is a comprehensive resource.

Vegan Challenge 22

challenge22.com

Let's Try Vegan: Get help with going vegan, including meal plans and support from registered dietitians. Sign up for free.

INSTAGRAM ACCOUNTS

Catherine, the Plant-Based RD

Instagram.com/plantbasedrd

Catherine is the queen of oatmeal bowls! You will find many delicious plant-based options on her feed. Catherine is a registered dietitian, so her advice is always science-based, and her recipes are healthy, beautiful, and easy.

Deliciously Ella

Instagram.com/deliciouslyella

Fun and healthy vegan recipes and lifestyle tips. This account, run by Ella Woodward, gives a UK perspective on healthy vegan recipes.

Dr. Matthew Nagra

Instagram.com/dr.matthewnagra

A naturopath with a solid grip on the data and a talent for communicating the info we all need, Dr. Nagra has a practice in Vancouver, Canada, and shares his knowledge of data in an accessible way.

Dr. Yami

Instagram.com/thedoctoryami

Dr. Yami Cazorla-Lancaster is a plant-based pediatrician who has a motivating style and great tips. Dr. Yami has a practice in Washington State, but she shares her knowledge with the vegan community via her social media and her podcast.

Lauren, Tasting to Thrive RD

Instagram.com/tastingtothrive_rd

Lauren offers delicious recipes and simple tips to improve your nutrition. She has such a warm and engaging style that you will find it easy to learn about plant-based nutrition just by following her account.

Lauren Toyota, Hot for Food

Instagram.com/hotforfood

Lauren has been active in the plant-based food movement since 2014 as a full-time blogger and YouTube personality. Check out her cookbooks, too: *Hot for Food: Vegan Comfort Classics* (Ten Speed Press, 2018) and *Hot for Food: All Day* (Ten Speed Press, 2021).

Lisa, the Viet Vegan

Instagram.com/thevietvegan

Here you'll find wonderful vegan recipes with a down-to-earth and friendly style. Learn to veganize your favorite Vietnamese recipes and get Lisa's delicious tofu egg salad recipe!

Plant-Proof

Instagram.com/plant_proof

Check out this Instagram account, podcast, and book for wonderful, science-based nutrition information. Based in Australia, this account is a good source of healthy vegan info for those living Down Under, or anywhere in the world.

REFERENCES

CHAPTER 1

Centers for Disease Control and Prevention. "Leading Causes of
Death." *FastStats.* Reviewed March 1, 2021. CDC.gov/nchs
/fastats/leading-causes-of-death.htm.

WebMD. "Insulin Resistance." Reviewed July 1, 2019. WebMD.com
/diabetes/insulin-resistance-syndrome.

CHAPTER 2

Alzheimer's Association. "2021 Alzheimer's Disease Facts and Fig-
ures." *Alzheimer's & Dementia* 17, no. 3 (2021). ALZ.org/media
/Documents/alzheimers-facts-and-figures.pdf.

American Cancer Society. "Infographic: Diet and Activity Guidelines to Reduce Cancer Risk." Accessed May 15, 2021. *Cancer
.Org*. Cancer.org/healthy/eat-healthy-get-active/acs-guidelines
-nutrition-physical-activity-cancer-prevention/infographic.html.

Appleby, Paul N., Gwyneth K. Davey, and Timothy J. Key. "Hypertension and Blood Pressure Among Meat Eaters, Fish Eaters,
Vegetarians and Vegans in EPIC–Oxford." *Public Health Nutrition* 5, no. 5 (2002): 645–54. DOI:10.1079/phn2002332.

Bouvard, Véronique, Dana Loomis, Kathryn Z. Guyton, Yann
Grosse, Fatiha El Ghissassi, Lamia Benbrahim-Tallaa, Neela
Guha, et al. "Carcinogenicity of Consumption of Red and
Processed Meat." *The Lancet Oncology* 16, no. 16 (2015):
1599–600. DOI:10.1016/s1470-2045(15)00444-1.

Centers for Disease Control and Prevention. "Facts About Hypertension." *High Blood Pressure*. Reviewed September 8, 2020.
CDC.gov/bloodpressure/facts.htm.

Centers for Disease Control and Prevention. *National Diabetes Statistics Report.* 2020. CDC.gov/diabetes/pdfs/data/statistics /national-diabetes-statistics-report.pdf.

Centers for Disease Control and Prevention. "Underlying Cause of Death, 1999–2019." *CDC Wonder.* Accessed May 15, 2021. *Wonder.CDC.gov.* Wonder.CDC.gov/ucd-icd10.html.

Esselstyn Jr., C. B., S. G. Ellis, S. V. Medendorp, and T. D. Crowe. "A Strategy to Arrest and Reverse Coronary Artery Disease: A 5-Year Longitudinal Study of a Single Physician's Practice." *Journal of Family Practice* 41, no. 6 (1995): 560–68.

Fraser, Gary, Sozina Katuli, Ramtin Anousheh, Synnove Knutsen, Patti Herring, and Jing Fan. "Vegetarian Diets and Cardiovascular Risk Factors in Black Members of the Adventist Health Study-2." *Public Health Nutrition* 18, no. 3 (2014): 537–45. DOI:10.1017/s1368980014000263.

Ghiasi, Shirin Sadat, Majid Jalalyazdi, Javad Ramezani, Azadeh Izadi-Moud, Fereshteh Madani-Sani, and Shokufeh Shahlaei. "Effect of Hibiscus Sabdariffa on Blood Pressure in Patients with Stage 1 Hypertension." *Journal of Advanced Pharmaceutical Technology & Research* 10, no. 3 (2019): 107. DOI:10.4103 /japtr.japtr_402_18.

Hales, C. M., M. D. Carroll, C. D. Fryar, and C. L. Ogden. "Prevalence of Obesity and Severe Obesity Among Adults: United States, 2017–2018." *NCHS Data Brief,* no. 360. National Center for Health Statistics. Reviewed February 27, 2020. CDC.gov/nchs /products/databriefs/db360.htm#ref1.

Hass, Ulrike, Catrin Herpich, and Kristina Norman. "Anti-Inflammatory Diets and Fatigue." *Nutrients* 11, no. 10 (2019): 2315. DOI:10.3390/nu11102315.

McMacken, Michelle, and Sapana Shah. "A Plant-Based Diet for the Prevention and Treatment of Type 2 Diabetes." *Journal of Geriatric Cardiology* 14, no. 5 (May 2017): 342–54. DOI.org/10.11909/j.issn.1671-5411.2017.05.009.

Mokdad, A., E. Ford, B. Bowman, D. Nelson, M. Engelgau, F. Vinicor, and J. Marks. "Diabetes Trends in the US: 1990–1998." *Diabetes Care*, 23, no. 9 (2000): 1278–83.

Morris, Martha Clare, Christy C. Tangney, Yamin Wang, Frank M. Sacks, David A. Bennett, and Neelum T. Aggarwal. "MIND Diet Associated with Reduced Incidence of Alzheimer's Disease." *Alzheimer's & Dementia* 11, no. 9 (2015): 1007–14. DOI:10.1016/j.jalz.2014.11.009.

Oh, Tae Jung, Jae Hoon Moon, Sung Hee Choi, Soo Lim, Kyong Soo Park, Nam H. Cho, and Hak Chul Jang. "Body-Weight Fluctuation and Incident Diabetes Mellitus, Cardiovascular Disease, and Mortality: A 16-Year Prospective Cohort Study." *Journal of Clinical Endocrinology & Metabolism* 104, no. 3 (2018): 639–46. DOI:10.1210/jc.2018-01239.

Pettersen, Betty J., Ramtin Anousheh, Jing Fan, Karen Jaceldo-Siegl, and Gary E. Fraser. "Vegetarian Diets and Blood Pressure Among White Subjects: Results from the Adventist Health Study-2 (AHS-2)." *Public Health Nutrition* 15, no. 10 (2012): 1909–16. DOI:10.1017/s1368980011003454.

Poirier, Abbey E., Yibing Ruan, Karena D. Volesky, Will D. King, Dylan E. O'Sullivan, Priyanka Gogna, Stephen D. Walter, et al. "The Current and Future Burden of Cancer Attributable to Modifiable Risk Factors in Canada: Summary of Results." *Preventive Medicine* 122 (2019): 140–47. DOI:10.1016/j.ypmed.2019.04.007.

Sarikaya, Hakan, Jose Ferro, and Marcel Arnold. "Stroke Prevention—Medical and Lifestyle Measures." *European Neurology* 73, nos. 3-4 (2015): 150–57. DOI:10.1159/000367652.

Viguiliouk, E., S. E. Stewart, V. H. Jayalath, A. P. Ng, A. Mirrahimi, R. J. de Souza, A. J. Hanley, et al. "Effect of Replacing Animal Protein with Plant Protein on Glycemic Control in Diabetes: A Systematic Review and Meta-Analysis of Randomized Controlled Trials." *Nutrients* 7, no. 12 (2015): 9804–24. DOI.org/10.3390/nu7125509.

Wharton, Sean, David C. W. Lau, Michael Vallis, Arya M. Sharma, Laurent Biertho, Denise Campbell-Scherer, Kristi Adamo, et al. "Obesity in Adults: A Clinical Practice Guideline." *Canadian Medical Association Journal* 192, no. 31 (2020): E875–91. DOI:10.1503/cmaj.191707.

CHAPTER 3

Brown, M. J. "Carotenoid Bioavailability Is Higher from Salads Ingested with Full-Fat Than with Fat-Reduced Salad Dressings as Measured with Electrochemical Detection." *American Journal of Clinical Nutrition* 80, no. 2 (August 2004): 396–403. DOI:10.1093/ajcn/80.2.396.

Butler, Stephanie. "Hoppin' John: A New Year's Tradition." *History*. Updated December 22, 2020. History.com/news/hoppin-john -a-new-years-tradition.

Cleveland Clinic. "6 Surprising Ways Garlic Boosts Your Health." *Health Essentials*. December 7, 2020. Health.ClevelandClinic .org/6-surprising-ways-garlic-boosts-your-health.

Dawson-Hughes, B. "Dietary Fat Increases Vitamin D-3 Absorption." *Journal of the Academy of Nutrition and Dietetics* 115, no. 2 (February 2015): 225–30. DOI:10.1016/j.jand.2014.09.014.

Graff, Rebecca E., Andreas Pettersson, Rosina T. Lis, Thomas U. Ahearn, Sarah C. Markt, Kathryn M. Wilson, Jennifer R. Rider, et al. "Dietary Lycopene Intake and Risk of Prostate Cancer Defined by ERG Protein Expression." *American Journal of Clinical Nutrition* 103, no. 3 (2016): 851–60. DOI:10.3945 /ajcn.115.118703.

Greger, Michael. "Dr. Greger's Daily Dozen." *NutritionFacts.org*. Accessed May 15, 2021. NutritionFacts.org/app/uploads/2018 /03/metric.png.

Harvard T. H. Chan School of Public Health. "Straight Talk About Soy." *The Nutrition Source*. Accessed May 15, 2021. HSPH .Harvard.edu/nutritionsource/soy.

Jacques, Paul F., Asya Lyass, Joseph M. Massaro, Ramachandran S. Vasan, and Ralph B. D'Agostino Sr. "Relationship of Lycopene Intake and Consumption of Tomato Products to Incident CVD." *British Journal of Nutrition* 110, no. 3 (2013): 545–51. DOI:10.1017/s0007114512005417.

Klemm, Sarah. "What Are Chia Seeds." *Eat Right.* Academy of Nutrition and Dietetics. Reviewed December 2020. EatRight.org/food/vitamins-and-supplements/nutrient-rich-foods/what-are-chia-seeds.

Kruse-Peeples, Melissa. "How to Grow a Three Sisters Garden." *Native Seeds Search.* May 27, 2016. NativeSeeds.org/blogs/blog-news/how-to-grow-a-three-sisters-garden.

Lock, Karen, Joceline Pomerleau, Louise Causer, Dan R. Altmann, and Martin McKee. "The Global Burden of Disease Attributable to Low Consumption of Fruit and Vegetables: Implications for the Global Strategy on Diet." *Bulletin of the World Health Organization* 83, no. 2 (February 2005): 81–160. WHO.int/bulletin/volumes/83/2/lock0205abstract/en.

National Institutes of Health, Office of Dietary Supplements. "Omega-3 Fatty Acids." US Department of Health and Human Services. Updated March 26, 2021. ODS.OD.NIH.gov/factsheets/Omega3FattyAcids-HealthProfessional.

National Peanut Board. "Peanut Per Capita Consumption Breaks New Record." September 8, 2020. NationalPeanutBoard.org/news/peanut-per-capita-consumption-breaks-new-record.htm.

PMA. "Top 20 Fruits and Vegetables Sold in the US." *The Packer.* Accessed May 15, 2021. PMA.com/content/articles/top-20-fruits-and-vegetables-sold-in-the-us.

Wu, Hongyu, Alan J. Flint, Qibin Qi, Rob M. van Dam, Laura A. Sampson, Eric B. Rimm, Michelle D. Holmes, et al. "Association between Dietary Whole Grain Intake and Risk of Mortality." *JAMA Internal Medicine* 175, no. 3 (2015): 373. DOI:10.1001/jamainternmed.2014.6283.

Wu, Xin, Jing Shi, Wan-xia Fang, Xiao-yu Guo, Ling-yun Zhang, Yun-peng Liu, and Zhi Li. "Allium Vegetables Are Associated with Reduced Risk of Colorectal Cancer: A Hospital-Based Matched Case-Control Study in China." *Asia-Pacific Journal of Clinical Oncology* 15, no. 5 (February 2019). DOI:10.1111/ajco.13133.

CHAPTER 4

Lappé, Frances Moore. *Diet for a Small Planet.* New York: Ballantine Books, 1971.

Mariotti, François, and Christopher D. Gardner. "Dietary Protein and Amino Acids in Vegetarian Diets—A Review." *Nutrients* 11, no. 11 (2019): 2661. DOI:10.3390/nu11112661.

Schaafsma, Gertjan. "The Protein Digestibility–Corrected Amino Acid Score." *Journal of Nutrition* 130, no. 7 (2000): 1865S–67S. DOI:10.1093/jn/130.7.1865s.

Thomas, D. Travis, Kelly Anne Erdman, and Louise M. Burke. "Position of the Academy of Nutrition and Dietetics, Dietitians of Canada, and the American College of Sports Medicine: Nutrition and Athletic Performance." *Journal of the Academy of Nutrition and Dietetics* 116, no. 3 (2016): 501–28. DOI:10.1016/j.jand.2015.12.006.

CHAPTER 5

Bilsborough, S. A., and T. C. Crowe. "Low-Carbohydrate Diets: What Are the Potential Short- and Long-Term Health Implications?" *Asia-Pacific Journal of Clinical Nutrition* 12, no. 4 (2003): 396–404. PMID: 14672862.

Harvard T. H. Chan School of Public Health. "Whole Grains." *Nutrition Source.* Accessed May 15, 2021. HSPH.Harvard.edu/nutritionsource/what-should-you-eat/whole-grains.

Holt, S. H., J. C. Miller, P. Petocz, and E. Farmakalidis. "A Satiety Index of Common Foods." *European Journal of Clinical Nutrition* 49, no. 9 (September 1995): 675–90. PMID: 7498104.

Tarray, Rayees, Sheikh Saleem, Dil Afroze, Irfan Yousuf, Azhara Gulnar, Bashir Laway, and Sawan Verma. "Role of Insulin Resistance in Essential Hypertension." *Cardiovascular Endocrinology* 3, no. 4 (2014): 129–33. DOI:10.1097/xce.0000000000000032.

USDA. *Dietary Guidelines for Americans 2020–2025*. December 2020. DietaryGuidelines.gov/sites/default/files/2020-12/Dietary_Guidelines_for_Americans_2020-2025.pdf.

Weickert, Martin O., and Andreas F. H. Pfeiffer. "Impact of Dietary Fiber Consumption on Insulin Resistance and the Prevention of Type 2 Diabetes." *Journal of Nutrition* 148, no. 1 (2018): 7–12. DOI:10.1093/jn/nxx008.

World Health Organization. "WHO Calls on Countries to Reduce Sugars Intake Among Adults and Children." March 4, 2015. WHO.int/news/item/04-03-2015-who-calls-on-countries-to-reduce-sugars-intake-among-adults-and-children.

CHAPTER 6

Danwatch. "How Much Water Does It Take to Grow an Avocado?" Accessed May 30. 2021. Old.Danwatch.dk/en/undersogelseskapitel/how-much-water-does-it-take-to-grow-an-avocado.

Guasch-Ferré, Marta, Gang Liu, Yanping Li, Laura Sampson, JoAnn E. Manson, Jordi Salas-Salvadó, Miguel A. Martínez-González, et al. "Olive Oil Consumption and Cardiovascular Risk in US Adults." *Journal of the American College of Cardiology* 75, no. 15 (2020): 1729–39. DOI:10.1016/j.jacc.2020.02.036.

Gunton, Jenny E., and Christian M. Girgis. "Vitamin D and Muscle." *Bone Reports* 8 (2018): 163–67. DOI:10.1016/j.bonr.2018.04.004.

Mozaffarian, Dariush, Renata Micha, and Sarah Wallace. 2021. "Effects on Coronary Heart Disease of Increasing Polyunsaturated Fat in Place of Saturated Fat: A Systematic Review and Meta-Analysis of Randomized Controlled Trials." *PLOS Medicine* 7 (March 2010): 1–10. DOI:10.1371/journal.pmed.1000252.

Neelakantan, Nithya, Jowy Yi Hoong Seah, and Rob M. van Dam. "The Effect of Coconut Oil Consumption on Cardiovascular Risk Factors." *Circulation* 141, no. 10 (2020): 803–14. DOI:10.1161/circulationaha.119.043052.

Pearce, Karma L., and Kelton Tremellen. "The Effect of Macronutrients on Reproductive Hormones in Overweight and Obese Men: A Pilot Study." *Nutrients* 11, no. 12 (2019): 3059. DOI:10.3390/nu11123059.

Ritchie, Hannah, and Max Roser. 2021. "Environmental Impacts of Food Production." *Our World in Data*. January 2020. OurWorldInData.org/environmental-impacts-of-food.

Sacks, Frank M., Alice H. Lichtenstein, Jason H. Y. Wu, Lawrence J. Appel, Mark A. Creager, Penny M. Kris-Etherton, Michael Miller, et al. "Dietary Fats and Cardiovascular Disease: A Presidential Advisory from the American Heart Association." *Circulation* 136 (June 15, 2017): e1–23. DOI:10.1161/cir.0000000000000510.

Schwingshackl, Lukas, and Georg Hoffmann. 2014. "Monounsaturated Fatty Acids, Olive Oil, and Health Status: A Systematic Review and Meta-Analysis of Cohort Studies." *Lipids in Health and Disease* 13, no. 1 (2014). DOI:10.1186/1476-511x-13-154.

Whittaker, Joseph, and Kexin Wu. "Low-Fat Diets and Testosterone in Men: Systematic Review and Meta-Analysis of Intervention Studies." *Journal of Steroid Biochemistry and Molecular Biology* 210 (2021): 105878. DOI:10.1016/j.jsbmb.2021.105878.

CHAPTER 7

Institute of Medicine. *Dietary Reference Intakes: The Essential Guide to Nutrient Requirements*. Washington, DC: the National Academies Press, 2006. DOI.org/10.17226/11537.

CHAPTER 8

Centers for Disease Control and Prevention. "Folic Acid." Last reviewed April 19, 2021. CDC.gov/ncbddd/folicacid/about.html.

Health Canada. "Do Canadian Children Meet Their Nutrient Requirements Through Food Intake Alone?" Government of Canada. 2012. Canada.ca/en/health-canada/services/food-nutrition/food-nutrition-surveillance/health-nutrition-surveys/canadian-community-health-survey-cchs/canadian-children-meet-their-nutrient-requirements-through-food-intake-alone-health-canada-2012.html.

Patel, Kushang V. "Epidemiology of Anemia in Older Adults." *Seminars in Hematology* 45, no. 4 (2008): 210–17. DOI:10.1053/j.seminhematol.2008.06.006.

Pfisterer, Kaylen J., Mike T. Sharratt, George G. Heckman, and Heather H. Keller. "Vitamin B_{12} Status in Older Adults Living in Ontario Long-Term Care Homes: Prevalence and Incidence of Deficiency with Supplementation as a Protective Factor." *Applied Physiology, Nutrition, and Metabolism* 41, no. 2 (2016): 219–22. DOI:10.1139/apnm-2015-0565.

CHAPTER 9

Melina, Vesanto, Winston Craig, and Susan Levin. "Position of the Academy of Nutrition and Dietetics: Vegetarian Diets." *Journal of the Academy of Nutrition and Dietetics* 116, no. 12 (2016): 1970–80. DOI:10.1016/j.jand.2016.09.025.

INDEX

D

Dairy alternatives, 38, 72
Dessert options, 117
Diabetes, 17–18. *See also*
    Insulin sensitivity
Diet for a Small Planet (Lappé), 49
Dining out, 110–111
Dinner options, 115–116
Dressing options, 118

E

Eat to Live (Fuhrman), 61
Energy, low, 109
Environmental benefits, 6–7
Esselstyn, Caldwell, Jr., 21, 79

F

Family support, 108
Fats
    about, 67–68
    children's nutritional needs, 95
    daily needs, 68–69
    and diabetes, 17
    and heart disease, 22
    monounsaturated, 73
    and muscle growth, 74
    polyunsaturated, 73
    saturated, 70
    sources of, 74–78
    trans, 73
    types of, 69–73
    unsaturated, 72–73
Fiber, 8, 63–65, 102
Flaxseed, 35, 76–77, 90
Folate, 98
Food labels, 40–41
Forks Over Knives (documentary), 21
Fortified foods, 90, 91
Friends support, 108
Fruits, 28–29
Fuhrman, Joel, 61

G

Gas and bloating, 109
Gelatin, 41
Grains. *See* Whole grains
Gut health, 7

H

Health at Every Size movement, 14–15
Health care providers, 108
Heart disease, 21–22
Herbs, 37
High blood pressure, 19
Honey, 38

I

Indian cuisine, 110
Inflammation, 15–16
Insulin sensitivity, 7–8, 62
Iodine
    about, 83–84
    children's nutritional needs, 96–97
    pregnancy and lactation
        needs, 99–100
Iron
    about, 84
    children's nutritional needs, 96
    older adults' nutritional needs, 102
    pregnancy and lactation needs, 98–99
    sources of, 99
Italian cuisine, 110

J

Japanese cuisine, 110

K

Kale, 31

L

Lactation, nutritional needs for, 98–101
Lactose, 41

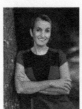

About the Author

PAMELA FERGUSSON has worked in nutrition for 20 years, both internationally and at home in Canada. She completed a master's and a PhD in nutrition, focusing on hunger and malnutrition in sub-Saharan Africa. Pamela then went on to work as a consultant for UNICEF and the World Food Program, and as a lecturer and researcher in the United Kingdom, the United States, and Canada.

Pamela has recently settled in the mountains of British Columbia with her four plant-based children: Bly, Cedar, Willow, and Fern. They love to cook vegan food and go skiing or hiking together. She runs a virtual private practice and consultancy firm from her home in Nelson, British Columbia.